NUTRITIONAL ASSESSMENT

A Manual for Practitioners

NUTRITIONAL ASSESSMENT

A Manual for Practitioners

Terri G. Jensen, R.D., M.S.
Consultant in Dietetics and Nutritional Support
Columbia, Missouri
Formerly, Coordinator of Surgical Nutrition
Hermann Hospital, and
Instructor, Department of Surgery
University of Texas Medical School in Houston

DeAnn Englert, R.N., M.S.
Consultant in Nutritional Support
Denver, Colorado
Formerly, TPN Nursing Coordinator
Hermann Hospital, and
Instructor, Department of Surgery
University of Texas Medical School in Houston

Stanley J. Dudrick, M.D., F.A.C.S.
Director of Nutritional Support Services
St. Luke's Episcopal Hospital, and
Professor of Surgery
University of Texas System Cancer Center
Houston, Texas

APPLETON-CENTURY-CROFTS/Norwalk, Connecticut

0-8385-7078-X

83 84 85 86 87 88 / 10 9 8 7 6 5 4 3 2 1

Prentice-Hall International, Inc., London
Prentice-Hall of Australia, Pty. Ltd., Sydney
Prentice-Hall Canada, Inc.
Prentice-Hall of India Private Limited, New Delhi
Prentice·Hall of Japan, Inc., Tokyo
Prentice-Hall of Southeast Asia (Pte.) Ltd., Singapore
Whitehall Books Ltd., Wellington, New Zealand
Editora Prentice-Hall do Brasil Ltda., Rio de Janeiro

Library of Congress Cataloging in Publication Data

Jensen, Terri G.
    Nutritional assessment.

    Bibliograpy: p.
    Includes index.
    1. Malnutrition.   2. Nutrition—Evaluation.   3. Diet
in disease.   I. Englert, DeAnn M.   II. Dudrick,
Stanley J.   III. Title.   [DNLM: 1. Nutrition.
2. Nutrition surveys.   3. Data collection— Methods.   QU 146.1
J54n]
RC623.J46   1983   616.3'9   82-24418
ISBN 0-8385-7078-X

Design: Jean M. Sabato

This book is dedicated to

Mrs. Jean Bottger, R.D., my source of
professional inspiration

and my parents
Mr. and Mrs. L.E. Gammeter

and family
Jack E. Jensen, M.D., Kristin and Justin

who have encouraged and supported my professional growth.

Contents

SECTION III
Guidelines for Interpreting
Nutritional Assessment Data

Preface

In 1976, a multidisciplinary nutritional assessment program was initiated at Hermann Hospital/The University of Texas Medical School in Houston, Texas, for the primary purposes of identifying patients with clinical and subclinical malnutrition, providing guidelines for nutritional care, and for evaluating patient response to subsequent nutritional therapy. Since that time, an increased awareness of the incidence and complications of hospital malnutrition and the advent of numerous sophisticated solutions and techniques for nutritional intervention have established the need for comprehensive nutritional assessment programs in many clinical situations. However, the implementation of such programs into traditional hospital settings presents a challenge to dietitians, physicians, and other health care professionals. Careful planning including definition of numerous procedures and development of forms for data collection and interpretation is essential for effective and successful implementation of nutritional assessment programs.

The intent of this manual is to provide the procedures and forms developed during the five-year operation of the nutritional assessment program at Hermann Hospital. The procedures for data collection contained herein have been used extensively to train dietitians, dietetic technicians, nutrition support nurses, and staff nurses in consistent and accurate initial and serial nutritional assessment data compilation. The guidelines for interpretation of nutritional assessment data include the clinical significance, standards and normal ranges and clinical considerations for accurate and consistent evaluation of nutritional status in hospitalized patients.

It is hoped that this manual will serve as a reference and guide for other professionals involved in the establishment of nutritional assessment programs. The definition of specific procedures for nutritional assessment is imperative to successful implementation and rapid growth of these programs.

Nutritional assessment is the rationale prerequisite to the provision of adequate nutritional support and should be a service available in all hospitals utilizing these techniques. It is encumbent upon health care professionals to interpret assimilated assessment data accurately while considering all possible clinical and biochemical variables if optimal nutrition is ever to be provided to all patients under all conditions at all times. It is a minor contribution to this ultimate goal that this book is written.

Terri G. Jensen, R.D., M.S.

Preface

Since the beginning of recorded medical history, physicians, scientists and other learned individuals, including Hippocrates, have noted that the prognosis for recovery from acute or chronic illnesses was poorer in persons with lean and slender bodies than in those who were well nourished. Thus, nutritional assessment had its origin as a series of empiric clinical observations and estimations of nutritional status, correlated with the ultimate results of diagnostic and therapeutic endeavors. Eventually a body of knowledge and experience developed which, coupled with logic and common sense, formed the basis for this very important aspect of clinical practice.

Consciously or unconsciously, physicians, surgeons and other health care personnel have been assessing the nutritional status of their patients for centuries in a variety of informal or formal ways as a means of helping them plan and execute the comprehensive management of their patients in order to predict the probable outcome of therapy. Although it may appear to some that nutritional assessment with its current resurgence of interest and emphasis is a relatively new aspect of health care and maintenance, standard medical examinations have routinely and for many decades included many important components for evaluating nutritional status. For example, a thoughtful and thorough history has included such nutritionally-related items as usual dietary intake and pattern, usual weight, maximum weight, recent weight change, food intolerance, gastrointestinal function, metabolic or endocrine disorders, exercise patterns, and so on. A physical examination would not be complete without noting the patient's vital signs, height and weight, skeletal development, body habitus, strength, somatic muscle mass and distribution, neuromuscular integrity, skin thickness and turgor, the presence or absence of the stigmata of deficiencies or excesses of specific nutrients or nutrient groups, etc. Even screening laboratory procedures have included urinalysis, complete blood count, chest x-ray, serum proteins, liver and kidney function tests, serum electrolytes, serum glucose and lipid concentrations, etc. More specific laboratory examinations have included evaluation of endocrine, gastrointestinal and other more complex metabolic functions.

The extent to which nutritional assessment is undertaken in each patient varies depending upon individual circumstances, and the judicious application of nutritional assessment techniques and methods requires some education, training, experience and good clinical judgment. Obviously, not all procedures are always applicable, nor should they be used uniformly in all patients. However, all patients should be assessed at least via a comprehensive history and physical examination and preferably with a standard set of screening criteria for evaluation, documentation and future comparison and reference. Only in this manner can objectivity be systematically obtained in an area in which subjectivity, with all of its vagaries, has been the rule in the past. When indicated, in-depth serial evaluations of nutritional status can be most helpful in appraising the patient's clinical course, documenting the effectiveness or ineffectiveness of therapy, indicating changes in therapeutic regimens, and predicting prognosis.

In special situations, study of the more complex indices of body composition, metabolism and immunocompetence may be indicated, and these procedures form the basis for the more sophisticated evaluation and analysis of nutritional status of the future. The development of low-cost automated biochemical and immunological serum microassays together with computerized integration of data will eventually allow the nutritional assessments of the past and present to advance and mature to the truly biochemical, metabolic and immunological assessments which will be commonplace in the future. It is anticipated that this will add an exciting scientific dimension to the understanding of the human organism in health and disease at a level heretofore not realized clinically. Until then, the authors hope that this manual will serve its intended purpose of providing a practical basis for understanding and applying the fundamentals of nutritional assessment for the primary goal of providing optimal nutrition to all patients under all conditions at all times.

Stanley J. Dudrick, M.D.

Acknowledgments _____

The Nutritional Assessment Manual was developed in conjunction with the Nutrition Support Team at Hermann Hospital. The authors greatly acknowledge the contributions of:

Betty Brooks, R.D., M.A., Cynthia Rapchack, B.S. Jeannie Flowers-Peas, B.S., Barbara Deverman, B.S., Cynthia Fanning, B.S., Belinda Garcia, B.S., Brian Rowlands, M.D., James Long, III, M.D., Chris Pacinda, R.N., Betsy Attaway, L.V.N., Patrick A. Mann, R.Ph.

Section I
Nutritional Assessment: General Information

A. Introduction

Nutritional assessment is a rational prerequisite to the provision of adequate patient care since virtually any disease, injury or surgical procedure can induce or intensify a state of clinical or subclinical malnutrition by altering nutrient ingestion, absorption, metabolism and/or requirements. Additionally, there is no known pathologic process from which a patient can be expected to recover better when he is malnourished than when he is well nourished.[1] Surveys of patients of varying socioeconomic backgrounds and differing diagnoses admitted to a variety of institutions have detected a high incidence of previously undocumented malnutrition, which once recognized may be corrected using a variety of nutritional support techniques.[2-8] In patients who exhibit signs, symptoms and/or history of malnutrition prior to hospitalization or who are likely to develop them during hospitalization as a result of stressful periods of diagnosis and treatment, a significantly higher morbidity and mortality can be expected if adequate attention is not directed to nutritional maintenance or restitution. Indeed, evidence has been reported to show that optimal results from surgical procedures, radiotherapy, chemotherapy, respiratory therapy and other forms of patient care can only be obtained when the patient is simultaneously in optimal nutritional condition.[9-15]

With the advent of numerous products, techniques and substrates which permit nutrient delivery and support to virtually every malnourished patient, the formerly inapparent or seemingly inevitable imbalances can now be corrected once they are identified. Therefore, not to nourish a patient adequately at this point in time reflects a positive decision to starve the patient or to passively accept starvation as the inevitable result.

Nutritional assessment is imperative to identify potential candidates for nutritional support, establish goals for nutritional intervention, delineate the most appropriate support modality and to evaluate serially the effectiveness of the prescribed therapy in ascertaining these goals. It is, therefore, anticipated that in the near future every health care facility will implement some type of routine nutritional assessment as part of the initial work-up and evaluation. The extent of this assessment will, of course, vary with the type of institution, the patient population and available manpower.

A multidisciplinary nutritional assessment program has been implemented by the Department of Dietetics in cooperation with the Department of Surgery and Nursing at Hermann Hospital/The University of Texas Medical School in Houston, Texas. The program has been operational for over 5 years and currently more than 100 patients are evaluated each day with comprehensive initial and serial nutritional assessments. The primary goal of this program is to provide meaningful nutritional data to the health care team throughout the entire course of patient care, from diagnosis through treatment, convalescence and rehabilitation. Secondary goals are to alert all health care professionals of the prevalence of malnutrition in hospitalized patients and to evaluate and delineate appropriate methods of clinical nutritional evaluation.

A variety of subjective and objective methods have been used in the clinical surveillance of hospitalized patients. This section presents a review of these methods and a discussion of their application and interpretation in clinical practice at Hermann Hospital.

B. Subjective Methods of Nutritional Assessment

Subjective data may be obtained by direct patient interview, through the medical history and nutrition history, and from the physical examination. Data derived directly from the patient can provide significant insight into the diagnosis and etiology of malnutrition. Additionally, because clinical variables influence the interpretation of objective data and eventual selection of nutrition support modalities, ongoing knowledge of subjective data is imperative.

MEDICAL HISTORY

Thorough review of the physician's medical history may identify numerous high-risk conditions that often occur concomitantly with malnutrition including hypermetabolic states, compromised digestive and absorptive capacity, chronic or acute diseases associated with abnormal nutrient intake or loss, recent major surgery and/or a treatment plan which has nutritional implications, i.e., chemotherapy. Since these situations are usually associated with nutritional depletion and related complications, the medical history provides a tool for identifying potential candidates for nutritional assessment and support.

PHYSICAL EXAMINATION

Adverse signs and symptoms of malnutrition are frequently documented in the physical examination and provide absolute indicators for further evaluation. These signs include hair changes—sparseness, dyspigmentation, and "pluckability"; skin changes—dermatitis, diffuse depigmentation, xerosis and follicular hyperkeratosis; confusion; apathy; parotid gland enlargement and hepatomegaly.[16] The most commonly recognized and documented signs of malnutrition are those which involve changes in body composition such as marked weight loss, loss of interosseous or supraclavicular musculature, or the presence of pitting edema, massive ascites or a scaphoid abdomen.[17] How-

related H. Failure — accumof serous fluid in peritoneal cavity   boat shaped

3

ever, these signs provide only a rough assessment of more extreme nutritional aberrations and are usually associated with very severe protein malnutrition. In the hospital, nutritional depletion often develops rapidly and becomes clinically significant before these signs appear. Although it is imperative to be cognizant of these signs in the malnourished patient and screen the physical examination for their occurrence, they are of little diagnostic value due to nonspecificity for malnutrition and their relatively late manifestation.

NUTRITION HISTORY

Additional subjective data of value in the diagnosis and treatment of malnutrition may be ascertained by direct patient interview. The nutrition history should focus on information which is consistent with nutritional risk such as recent changes in weight, appetite and food intake. Other useful information which can be gleaned from this interview include food aversions, intolerances, and/or difficulties with mastication or deglutition which are useful in planning subsequent care. After the purpose of the nutrition history in the total nutritional assessment scheme is established, key questions can be identified to elicit desired information (Table 1).

TABLE 1. KEY QUESTIONS—DIRECT PATIENT INTERVIEW

Present height and weight
Usual weight
Maximum weight and date
Changes in weight
Changes in appetite
Changes in food intake
Special diet at home
Elimination pattern
Nausea and vomiting
Food aversions, intolerances and allergies
Mechanical feeding problems
Medications and nutrition supplements
Occupation and usual daily activity
Usual energy and nutrient intake (24-hour recall)

C. Objective Methods of Nutritional Assessment

Anthropometric measurements (height, weight, triceps skinfold thickness and midupper arm circumference), biochemical testing (creatinine/height index, serum albumin, serum transferrin, serum prealbumin, retinol-binding protein, nitrogen balance, total lymphocyte count) and recall skin antigen testing are objective methods of nutritional assessment which are currently widely used in clinical practice. These measurements and tests provide a gross quantitative evaluation of tissue composition as well as an estimate of endogenous stores that are available to satisfy energy requirements. In addition, objective data is used to formulate appropriate nutritional regimens and document the efficacy of selected therapeutic intervention.

WEIGHT

Body weight is the most widely used index of nutritional status and is a valuable general indicator of malnutrition. Additionally, weight change is a relatively simple but valuable indicator of nutritional risk and rehabilitation when weights are measured accurately and regularly with sufficient knowledge of all active clinical and biochemical variables. A platform balance scale is usually used to measure body weight in the hospital (see Section II-D). Patients who cannot assume an upright stance for weighing on a platform balance scale can be weighed using a wheelchair scale, bed scale or lift bed scale (see Section II-E).

The percent ideal body weight, percent usual weight and percent weight change over a defined period of time can then be calculated to provide clinically useful information.[18] These data provide an indication of the need for nutritional intervention, and daily recorded weights are of value in the assessment of fluid balance and response to therapy (see Section III-A).

5

HEIGHT

Height is measured to provide an index for comparison of weight and/or creatinine excretion determinations with published standards. Stature (standing height) is defined as the distance from the sole of the feet to the top of the head and is measured with a vertical rod or measuring tape while the patient is standing erect so that the line of sight is horizontal and the heels and scapulae are aligned (see Section II-C). If the patient is unable to assume this position, height can be measured with a tape measure in the supine position or the clinician can rely on patient history.

TRICEPS SKINFOLD

Fat, somatic tissue protein and visceral protein are the three major body tissues that are available to meet the energy requirements of the catabolic patient and critical analysis of these components are essential to validate interpretations of body weight. Adipose tissue, the primary caloric reserve of the body, is assessed by measuring the triceps skinfold which includes the subcutaneous fat layer. Although 22 body sites have been documented for the measurement of skinfold thickness, the triceps area is most commonly measured since standards are available for the American population. Precise measurement technique is mandatory because the fat distribution in the upper arm is not uniform and limitations in accuracy depend primarily on location of the skinfold and intraobserver variability (see Sections II-F and II-H). Utilization of defined procedures may be impossible in patients with orthopedic, neurologic, burn and other injuries who are unable to sit or stand upright because of limitations imposed by traction, mental status, massive injury or other common impediments. In these instances the triceps skinfold can be measured accurately, reproducibly and comparably in the supine position with minor alterations in procedure (see Section II-G).

p. 79

ARM CIRCUMFERENCE

The status of skeletal muscle mass or somatic protein can be estimated by calculating arm muscle circumference and arm muscle area. These measurements are commonly depressed during chronic protein and energy deprivation as skeletal muscle is catabolized to provide energy substrate. The arm muscle circumference and area are derived from measurements of triceps skinfold and arm circumference (see Sections II-F and II-G). Initial measurements are compared to published standards to indicate the degree of somatic tissue depletion and to serial determinations to indicate comparative changes in skeletal muscle protein during nutritional repletion, although limitations of anthropometric measurements must be considered in data interpretation (see Section III-B).

CREATININE/HEIGHT INDEX

The creatinine/height index provides another estimate of skeletal muscle mass since urinary levels of creatinine are dependent principally upon the extent of skeletal muscle catabolism, particularly during

NUTRITION   QUESTIONNAIRE
HERMANN HOSPITAL/THE UNIVERSITY HOSPITAL

PLEASE COMPLETE: 1 - 15

1. What is the most you have weighed? _____ When? _____

2. Has your weight recently changed? ☐ Yes (☐ Lost ☐ Gained) ☐ No

   How much? _____ When? _____

3. Do you follow a special diet at home? ☐ Yes ☐ No

   If yes, please specify type _____

DATE OF SERVICE

4. Are there any foods you deliberately avoid? ☐ Yes ☐ No

   If yes, please specify what and why _____

5. Do you have any food intolerances or allergies? ☐ Yes ☐ No

   If yes, please specify _____

6. Have you recently experienced ☐ Nausea ☐ Vomiting ☐ Diarrhea ☐ Constipation ☐ Other _____

7. Do you have any chewing or swallowing problems? ☐ Yes ☐ No

   If yes, please specify _____

8. Have you experienced any recent changes in your appetite? ☐ Yes ☐ No

   If yes, please specify _____

9. Has your food intake recently increased? ☐ Yes ☐ No   Decreased? ☐ Yes ☐ No

   If yes, please specify _____

10. Are you taking any vitamins or nutritional supplements? ☐ Yes ☐ No

    If yes, please specify what kind _____

11. What is your occupation? _____

12. Are you being treated for any disease? ☐ Yes ☐ No

    If yes, list problems and medications _____

13. Have you ever had an operation? ☐ Yes ☐ No

    If yes, please specify operation and date _____

14. Have you ever had mumps? ☐ Yes ☐ No   Tuberculosis? ☐ Yes ☐ No

15. Is there anything that you feel is important for the dietitian to know in planning your nutritional care? _____

(continued)

Figure 1. Nutrition Questionnaire.

Please write below everything you eat on a normal day, include snacks, and beverages. Begin with the first thing you eat or drink when you get up in the morning. Please let us know what you season your foods with as salt, pepper, butter, etc.

TIME	FOOD	HOW MUCH?	FOR DIETITIANS USE

		CALORIES	CHO	PRO	FAT
Average daily calorie intake (History)		_____	_____	_____	_____

Figure 1. *Continued.*

protein depletion. The creatinine/height index is defined as the 24-hour creatinine excretion of a patient divided by the expected 24-hour creatinine excretion of a normal adult of the same height.[18] Determination of the creatinine/height index, therefore, requires collection of an accurate 24-hour urine specimen for analysis (see Section II-M). The creatinine/height index is a very sensitive measure of not only muscle mass, but work tolerance. Physical activity and other factors must be considered in the interpretation of data (see Section III-C).

SERUM PROTEINS

The degree of visceral protein depletion is estimated by determining serum concentrations of albumin, transferrin, prealbumin and/or retinol-binding protein. Serum albumin levels fall only after significant protein depletion has occurred. Serum albumin is usually measured by an adaption of the Bromcresol Green (BCG) dye-binding method, which is recognized to be superior to other dye-binding techniques because of its specificity and freedom from interference. Serum transferrin is a more sensitive indicator of marginal protein depletion because of its shorter half-life of eight days. Serum transferrin is measured by the radial immunodiffusion technique of Mancini, which in our experience is a more accurate assessment of visceral protein status than indirect derivation from serum total iron binding capacity.[19] Retinol-binding protein and prealbumin have also been shown to be sensitive indicators of visceral protein status and are depressed before transferrin due to their even shorter half-lives of 12 hours and 48 hours respectively.[20] Serum retinol-binding protein and prealbumin concentrations are also easily quantitated by radial immunodiffusion (see Section II-L). Serum protein concentrations reflect nutritional rehabilitation effectively. However, factors other than catabolism, such as excretion, intravascular change, interstitial transfer and state of hydration, may influence plasma concentrations (see Sections III-D, E and F).

NITROGEN BALANCE

Since nitrogen is the primary component that differentiates protein from other basic nutrient moieties, and since protein status reflects the overall state of nutrition, nitrogen balance is also employed as an index of protein nutritional status. Because urea accounts for approximately 90 percent of total urinary nitrogen loss, nitrogen balance can be computed for clinical purposes from measurement of urine urea nitrogen as nitrogen intake minus (UUN + 4). The latter factor accounts for stool and skin losses as well as nonurea urinary nitrogen loss.[18] While less precise than other methods, this formula provides an inexpensive, clinically applicable working estimate of nitrogen balance and can serve as a valuable guide to the adequacy of nutritional support (see Section III-G).

TOTAL LYMPHOCYTE COUNT

absence of Rx to a specific antigen or allergen

In anergic patients, the total lymphocyte count is often reduced by as much as one-third. Although lymphopenia can be induced by numerous clinical stresses such as radiation therapy and halothane anesthesia, it is most commonly secondary to malnutrition. Nutritional repletion can correct lymphopenia despite continuation of the disease process (see Section III-H).

SKIN ANTIGEN TESTING

Loss of immunocompetence is another indication of visceral protein depletion and is strongly correlated with malnutrition. Protein malnutrition is associated with impaired host defense mechanisms, particularly cell-mediated immunity as manifested by recall skin antigen testing. One-tenth ml of trychophyton, Candida®, streptokinase/streptodornase, mumps and intermediate purified protein derivative (PPD) are injected into the dermis of the volar aspect of the forearm, and the reactions are measured at 24 and 48 hours following injection (see Sections II-N, II-O, II-P and III-I).

D. Indications for Nutritional Assessment: Screening _____

Definite indications for nutritional assessment and support include those patients with suspected protein and/or calorie undernutrition, those with hypermetabolic illnesses and injuries, those who are unable or unwilling to eat, and those with specific diseases requiring nutritional therapy. In these instances, comprehensive nutritional evaluation is considered essential to proper patient management.

All patients with suspected protein and/or calorie undernutrition are identified by a screening nutritional assessment performed soon after admission to the hospital (see Section II-A). This assessment utilizes selected demographic, subjective, anthropometric and laboratory data which are collected routinely during admission to the hospital. Within 48 hours after admission to the hospital, the medical record is reviewed to determine the patient's height, weight, age, sex, initial diagnosis, serum albumin concentration, white blood cell count and differential for lymphocytes. The patient is interviewed to ascertain his usual weight and the date this weight was last recorded. The presence of gastrointestinal signs and symptoms which are consistent with nutritional depletion, i.e., nausea, vomiting, diarrhea, dysphagia and/or abdominal pain, are also noted. At this time, the triceps skinfold thickness and arm circumference are measured and recorded. All data are then typed into a computer and a profile of output data is generated which graphically depicts the need for further evaluation and support. The percent ideal weight, percent usual weight, percent weight change and percentage of standard for anthropometric measurements are calculated and recorded. A complete nutritional profile is recommended if the patient is less than 80 percent of ideal weight, reports a recent unintentional weight loss of greater than 10 pounds, has triceps skinfold or arm circumference measurements less than 80 percent of standard, has a serum albumin concentration of less than 3.5 g/dl, and/or a total lymphocyte count of less than 1500 cells/cu mm. Additionally, a history of change in appetite or food intake, nausea, vomiting, diarrhea or recent surgery indicate potential nutritional risk and a comprehensive profile is recommended.

In addition to those patients identified by the above screening procedures, a complete nutrition profile is automatically ordered for those patients admitted with multiple trauma, sepsis, long-bone fracture and second- or third-degree burns. These hypermetabolic states are usually associated with nutritional depletion and related complications as a result of reduced nutrient intake and greatly increased nutrient requirements. In these cases, screening evaluation is unnecessary and a comprehensive nutritional assessment is automatically commenced when the patient is hemodynamically stable and is in normal acid-base and fluid and electrolyte balance.

Comprehensive assessment is also ordered automatically for those patients admitted with diagnoses commonly associated with an inability to eat or who should not eat because of the nature of their disease processes. Patients who cannot eat include those with esophageal carcinoma, achalasia, gastric carcinoma, obstructing peptic ulcer, superior mesenteric artery syndrome, paralytic ileus, obstructing colonic carcinoma, malabsorption syndrome, peritonitis and obstructing diverticulitis. Patients who are not allowed to eat include those with enterocutaneous or enteroenteric fistulas, acute inflammatory bowel disease and acute pancreatitis. Patients admitted for chemotherapy and radiation therapy, or with chronic renal or hepatic disease are often nutritionally depleted and therefore complete nutritional assessment is automatically obtained.

E. Comprehensive Nutritional Assessment _____

Comprehensive nutritional assessment is ordered to classify further the type and degree of malnutrition and to identify the etiology (see Section II-B). Data obtained from this assessment provide guidelines for planning nutrition care and evaluating patient response to therapy.

The protocol for comprehensive nutritional assessment requires the collection of additional objective and subjective data. A complete dietary history is obtained using 24-hour recall techniques to evaluate the adequacy of previous nutrient intake. Additional interview questions relate to medications, food aversions, intolerances, allergies or difficulties with mastication and deglutition. Occupational and other physical activities are evaluated and correlated with an assessment of energy expenditure. Energy requirements are calculated as the sum basal energy expenditure (BEE), the calories consumed for physical activity, the specific dynamic action of food and increased energy requirements for sepsis, fever, trauma, disease and surgery. Basal energy expenditure is calculated from the Harris-Benedict equation, which is based on the age, sex, height and weight of the patient.[21] A 10 percent increase above basal rates is calculated for those patients who are confined to bed and the majority of ambulatory patients expend no more than 20 percent above basal rates for physical activity during hospitalization.[22] The specific dynamic action of food is calculated as approximately 10 percent of orally or enterally consumed calories. Approximate values for the increase in basal energy expenditure above normal levels during injury and stress have been established utilizing gas exchange and nitrogen excretion measurements in surgical patients and are used to estimate total energy requirements.[23,24] These increases in BEE may range from 10 percent in a patient undergoing elective surgery without complications to 125 percent above predicted values following major thermal injury. Protein requirements are then estimated using the formula:

$$\text{Protein (g)} = \frac{6.25 \times \text{energy requirements}}{150}$$

A nonprotein calorie to nitrogen ratio of 150:1 is adequate for most catabolic patients although the ratio may be adjusted in cases of renal disease, hepatic dysfunction, hypoproteinemic obesity or severe stress. Evaluation of each patient's unique circumstances thus permits an initial estimate of energy and protein requirements. Based on this assessment, nutritional therapy is initiated but may subsequently be altered in accordance with changes in the patient's clinical condition.

In addition to data collected for screening purposes, supplemental data collected for comprehensive nutritional assessment include serum transferrin, serum prealbumin, serum retinol-binding protein, and 24-hour urine urea nitrogen and creatinine excretion for computation of nitrogen balance and creatinine/height index. A battery of five skin test antigens (trychophytin, purified protein derivative (PPD), mumps, Candida and streptokinase-streptodornase) is applied to evaluate cell-mediated immunity and immunocompetence.

F. Serial Assessment

Each objective test, measurement and calculation is repeated serially every 10 days to assess the patient's response to nutritional therapy. A complete nutrition profile summarizing all nutrition data is generated and submitted to the medical record every 12 days. Body weights and energy/nutrient intakes from oral, enteral and parenteral sources are monitored and recorded daily. The percentage of weight change since admission and since the last assessment is calculated to provide an ongoing evaluation of progress. Average caloric and protein intakes are also computed every 10 days to indicate appropriate adjustments in nutritional therapy.

G. Assimilation of Nutritional Assessment Data _____

The collection and assimilation of the aforementioned data requires a full-time commitment of specially trained nutrition technicians and a major commitment from staff nurses, nutrition support nurses, clinical dietitians and physicians. Careful coordination of their individual program activities is essential and is achieved by a secretarial coordinator.

NUTRITION TECHNICIANS

Utilization of support personnel is essential to extend nutritional assessment services to large numbers of hospitalized and ambulatory patients while freeing the dietitian to assume other professional responsibilities. The nutrition technicians employed in the nutritional assessment program at Hermann Hospital have successfully completed a Bachelor of Science degree in Dietetics and Nutrition or an associate degree program which meets educational standards established by the American Dietetics Association for dietetic technician status. In addition, they must demonstrate a minimum entry level of competency designated in a training manual at the conclusion of a three-week training course.

The nutrition technicians are responsible for all data collection for screening nutritional assessment (see Section II-A). After obtaining a daily list of new admissions, they review the medical record for routine admission demographic data and laboratory results and interview the patient for specific subjective information relating to usual weight and gastrointestinal symptoms consistent with nutritional aberrations. The nutrition technicians also perform anthropometric measurements for screening, comprehensive and serial nutritional assessments (see Sections II-C, II-F and II-G). Nutrition technicians collect daily oral, enteral and parenteral intake records, calculate actual daily intakes and record this information, along with daily weights, in the medical record, under the direct supervision of the clinical dietitian (see Sections II-I and II-K). Additionally, a general order set for nutritional assessment has enabled the nutrition technicians to order initial and serial laboratory tests and has ensured the timely collection of specimens (see Section II-L). Serial assessment involves the coordination of activities for skin testing, laboratory testing, urine collection, anthropometric measurements and the recording of nutrient intakes at regular intervals. The nutrition technician is responsible for scheduling these activities to ensure that all data are collected according to protocol. The nutrition technician, when fully knowledgeable of the procedures for nutritional evaluation, may also participate in orientation and inservice programs. These sessions, which emphasize the purposes of the program and the patient benefits, facilitate understanding and acceptance of the program by all professionals involved in patient care. Procedures for urine collection, skin testing, daily weights and recording food and fluid intakes must be reinforced periodically. The technicians use audiovisual instruction, hand-outs and individual instruction based on specific procedures to facilitate mastery of these procedures among all professionals involved (see Section II). Working in this capacity, each technician is responsible for a maximum of 30 patients who are undergoing comprehensive assessment.

STAFF NURSES

Staff nurses collect 24-hour urine samples, measure and record daily weights, and record 24-hour enteral food, fluid and formula intakes on designated record sheets. Parenteral infusate is recorded on specific records and in the input and output section of the nursing notes (see Sections II-D, II-E, II-J and II-M).

NUTRITION SUPPORT NURSES

Nutrition support nurses are notified to administer recall skin test antigens initially and serially every 10 days and are also responsible for reading and interpreting the results at 24 and 48 hours postinjection. Any adverse reaction or problem is charted by the nurse at the time of administration or reading (see Sections II-N, II-O and II-P).

SECRETARIAL COORDINATOR

All incoming data from nutrition technicians, staff nurses, nutrition support nurses and laboratory representatives are assimilated on a specific data record and entered into a WANG 2000 model computer through a programmed Aimes Software package by the secretarial coordinator. The Nutritional Assessment Center functions as the central unit for processing incoming data, housing equipment and patient files, and offices the secretarial coordinator and nutrition technicians.

Charges for nutritional assessment services are also generated and processed in the Nutritional Assessment Center by the secretarial coordinator. A fee of $115.00 is charged for collection, assimilation and interpretation of data for the initial comprehensive assessment and for every serial assessment thereafter. The screening assessment is performed at no additional cost to the patient. The income is utilized to cover labor and material costs incurred for services rendered. At present, four nutrition technicians' and the secretarial coordinator's salaries are paid through this cost center. Additional costs are incurred for forms, equipment and computer rental. Blue Cross/Blue Shield of Texas has granted third party reimbursement for these services.

The secretarial coordinator is also responsible for ordering supplies and scheduling the technicians. The secretarial coordinator assimilates and organizes output graphs and charts for interpretation by professional team members and prepares them for submission to the medical record. Additionally, she schedules rounds and case conferences in the center to enhance communication of results and indicated modifications in nutrition care among professional and support personnel.

CLINICAL DIETITIANS

Clinical dietitians are responsible for interpreting assimilated data, assessing individual nutrient requirements, developing, implementing and evaluating indicated nutritional care plans and communicating nutritional assessment data. Each patient is interviewed by a clinical dietitian within 72 hours after comprehensive nutritional assessment is ordered to obtain subjective data and to estimate protein and energy requirements.

Because the clinical dietitian is specifically trained and educated to interpret anthropometric, biochemical and other data relative to nutritional status, a primary responsibility is to assist with cautious interpretation of data considering interrelated clinical factors which may influence readings and results of tests used. Recommendations for nutrition care are made by the dietitian based on estimated nutrient requirements, the interpretation of nutritional assessment data and on the patient's ability to tolerate various forms of nutrition therapy. Nutrient intakes, serial objective data and subjective assessment of the patient's tolerance of therapy are recorded by the dietitian in the medical record along with recommendations for changes in nutritional care. In addition to writing admission, progress and discharge notes in the medical record, participation on formal and informal rounds ensures effective communication of data on a daily basis.

The daily operation of the nutritional assessment program is supervised by the coordinator of nutrition services, a clinical dietitian who is knowledgeable in all clinical and administrative aspects of the program. The coordinator is responsible for supervising all aspects of data collection, assimilation and interpretation and for training and evaluating nutrition technicians and dietitians according to established procedures.

PHYSICIAN

The physician contributes clinical expertise in the science of nutrition and the techniques for enteral and parenteral nutritional support. The physician contributes knowledge of the patient's disease process, clinical course and treatment plan and notes the effects of disease, operative procedures and medications on interpretation of the results. The physicians working in this program are faculty general surgeons who are particularly interested and skilled in nutritional evaluation and therapy. However, other physicians may become involved in the team's activities by ordering nutritional assessment of their patients and by discussing the management of patients requiring nutritional support with established team members.

H. Interpretation of Nutritional Assessment Data

Protein-calorie malnutrition may be divided into three major classifications based on pathogenesis and clinical findings.

Kwashiorkor is common in patients with a combination of severe catabolic stress and low protein intake. The patients often maintain normal anthropometric measurements while visceral protein mass is significantly depleted and circulating protein levels are depressed together with the cellular immune system.

Marasmus is a chronic illness characterized by gradual wasting of somatic protein mass and subcutaneous fat reserves due to inadequate consumption of both calories and protein. This leads to impairment of vital muscular functions and tissue healing, and immune function becomes depressed as the severity of the disease increases.

Marasmus-kwashiorkor is a state of severe nutritional depletion characterized by the features of both marasmus and kwashiorkor, leading to the depletion of body fat, somatic and visceral protein.

The above diagnoses are identified in the International Classification of Diseases, however, combinations and degrees of each exist. The depression of any index or measurement may substantiate the need for aggressive nutritional intervention when considered with the patient's history, clinical course and treatment plan. Careful consideration of the patient's clinical condition, nutrient requirements and clinical treatment is therefore essential for valid interpretation of data. Serum protein levels and skin test responses may be temporarily altered by sepsis, medications, surgery or traumatic episodes. All possible clinical and biochemical variables must be considered if optimal nutrition is to be provided (see Section III).

REFERENCES

1. Dudrick, S.J. and Duke, J.H. Jr.: Nutritional complications in the surgical patient, in Complications in Surgery and Their Management, 3rd edition. Artz, C.P. and Hardy, J.D. (eds), Philadelphia: W.B. Saunders, 1975, pp. 243-276.

2. Hill, G.L., Blacket, R.L., et al.: Malnutrition in Surgical Patients: An Unrecognized Problem. Lancet 1:689, 1977.
3. Weinsier, R.L., Hunker, E.M., et al.: Hospital malnutrition: A prospective evaluation of general medicine patients during the course of hospitalization. Am. J. Clin. Nutr. 32:418, 1979.
4. Willard, M.D. Protein-calorie malnutrition in a community hospital. JAMA 243:1720, 1980.
5. Bistrian, B.R., Blackburn, G.L., et al.: Protein status of general surgical patients. JAMA 230:850, 1974.
6. Bistrian, B.R., Blackborn, G.L., et al.: Prevalence of malnutrition in general medical patients. JAMA 235:1567, 1976.
7. Reinhardt, G.F., Myscofski, J.W., et al.: Incidence of hypoalbuminemia in a hospitalized veteran population. JPEN 4:81, 1980 (Abstr).
8. Bollot, A.J. and Owens, S.D.: Evaluation of nutritional status of selected hospitalized patients. Am. J. Clin. Nutr. 26:931, 1973.
9. Kaminski, M.V., Fitzgerald, M.T., et al.: Correlation of mortality with serum transferrin and anergy. JPEN 1:27, 1977.
10. MacLean, L.D., Meakins, J.L., et al.: Host resistance in sepsis and trauma. Ann. Surg. 182:207, 1975.
11. Rhoads, J.E. and Alexander, C.E.: Nutritional problems in surgical patients. Ann. N.Y. Acad. Sci. 63:268, 1955.
12. Lewis, T.R. and Klein, H.: Risk factors in postoperative sepsis: Significance of preoperative lymphocytopenia. J. Surg. Re. 26:365, 1979.
13. Mullen, J.L., Gertner, M.H., et al.: Implications of malnutrition in the surgical patient. Arch. Surg. 114:121, 1979.
14. Thompson, W.D.: Effect of hypoproteinemia on wound disruption. Arch. Surg. 36:500, 1978.
15. Copeland, E.M. and Dudrick, S.J.: Nutritional aspects of cancer, in Current Problems in Cancer. Hickey, R.C. (ed), Chicago: Year Book Medical Publishers, Inc., 1976.
16. Cristakis, G.: Nutritional Assessment in Health Programs. Washington, D.C.: American Public Health Association, Inc., 1974.
17. Dudrick, S.J., Jensen, T.G., and Rowlands, B.J.: Nutrition support: Assessment and indications, in Nutrition in Clinical Surgery. Dietel M. (ed), Baltimore: Williams and Wilkins, 1980, pp. 13-18.
18. Blackburn, G.L., Bistrian, B.R., et al.: Nutritional and metabolic assessment of the hospitalized patient. JPEN 1:11, 1979.
19. Rowlands, B.J., Jensen, T.G. and Dudrick, S.J.: Comparison of two methods for measurement of serum transferrin. JPEN 3:504, 1979.
20. Shetty, P.S., Jung, R.J., et al.: Rapid turnover transport proteins: An index of subclinical protein-energy malnutrition. Lancet 2:230, 1979.
21. Harris, J.A. and Benedict, F.G.: A biometric study of basal metabolism in man. Carnegie Institution of Washington, Publication No. 279, Washington, 1919.
22. Kinney, J.M.: Energy requirements of the surgical patient, in Manual of Surgical Nutrition. Ballinger, W.F., Collins, J.A., Drucker, J.A., et al. (eds), Philadelphia: W.B. Saunders, 1979, pp. 223-235.
23. Kinney, J.M., Long, C.L., et al.: Tissue composition of weight loss in surgical patients: Elective operation. Ann. Surg. 168:459, 1968.
24. Long, C.L., Schaffel, N., et al.: Metabolic response to injury and illness: Estimation of energy and protein needs by indirect calorimetry and nitrogen balance. JPEN 3:452, 1979.

Section II
Nutritional Assessment Procedures: Data Collection

A. Procedure for Screening Nutritional Assessment

PURPOSE

The purposes of the procedure for screening nutritional assessment are:

1. To identify patients with subjective and/or objective evidence of nutritional depletion within 48 hours after admission to the hospital.
2. To provide guidelines for initiation of comprehensive serial nutritional assessment and subsequent nutrition therapy.

GENERAL INFORMATION

1. Patients admitted to the hospital will be nutritionally assessed by screening evaluation procedure within 24 hours after admission to the hospital unless comprehensive nutritional assessment is ordered.
2. Patients with diagnoses of burns and multiple trauma will not be screened since these hypermetabolic states are associated with nutritional depletion as a result of injury and increased energy and nutrient requirements. Comprehensive nutritional assessment will automatically be instituted on the fifth postinjury day in these cases.
3. Data for screening nutritional assessment will be collected by nutrition technicians from the Department of Dietetics, Nutritional Assessment Program.
4. No additional laboratory testing is required for screening nutritional assessment since the laboratory tests utilized are automatically ordered at admission for all patients admitted to surgery services.
5. All data for screening nutritional evaluation will be interpreted by a registered clinical dietitian.
6. The completed Screening Nutrition Profile will be submitted to the progress notes of the medical record within 48 hours after admission to the hospital.

SCREENING NUTRITIONAL ASSESSMENT
DATA CARD
The Hermann Hospital / The University Hospital

Demographic Data	Objective Data
Name _____	Serum Albumin _____ g/dl
Room # _____	WBC _____ cells/mm^3
Hospital # _____	Lymphocytes _____ %
Physician _____	Weight _____ lb
Service _____	Height _____ in.
Admission Date _____	Triceps Skinfold _____ mm
Diagnosis _____	Arm Circumference _____ cm
Sex _____ Age _____ yr. _____	

Subjective Data

Usual Weight _____ lb.   Date Last Recorded _____

☐ **Nausea**   ☐ Vomiting   ☐ Diarrhea   ☐ Dysphagia   ☐ Abdominal Pain
☐ **Other**

_____
Signature

Figure 1. Screening Nutritional Assessment Data Card. All data collected to screen patients for nutritional aberrations are recorded on this card.

EQUIPMENT

- Platform balance scale or bed scale
- Lange skinfold caliper
- Insertion measurement tape
- Pen or pencil
- Screening Nutritional Assessment Data Card

PROCEDURE

1. Within 24 hours after new patients are admitted to the hospital, a nutrition technician or clinical dietitian will review the patient's medical record and record the following on the Screening Nutritional Assessment Data Card (Fig. 1).
   a. Patient name and room number.
   b. Hospital identification number.
   c. Attending physician and service.
   d. Admission date.
   e. Admitting diagnosis and/or chief complaint.
   f. Age and sex.
   g. Serum albumin concentration.
   h. White blood cell count.
   i. Differential for lymphocytes.
   (*Note:* If laboratory test results have not been recorded in the medical record, the nutrition technician will call the chemistry laboratory and request these results.)
2. The nutrition technician or clinical dietitian will explain the purpose of the screening assessment procedure to the patient, ascertain the following information and record on the data card:
   a. Usual weight.
   b. Date the usual weight was last recorded (approximate).

    c. Recent history of nausea, vomiting, diarrhea, dysphagia and / or abdominal pain.

3. The nutrition technician or staff nurse will weigh and measure the patient using a platform balance scale and record weight in pounds and height in inches on the Screening Nutritional Assessment Data Card (see Sections II-C and II-D). If a bed scale is required to weigh the patient, the nutrition technician will notify the primary nurse to weigh the patient (see Section II-E).

4. The nutrition technician will obtain three measurements of triceps skinfold and arm circumference and record the average measurements on the Screening Nutritional Assessment Data Card (see Sections II-F and II-G).

5. The completed Screening Nutritional Assessment Data Card will be signed and submitted to the Nutritional Assessment Center by the nutrition technician. The name and room number of any patient who can not be evaluated for any reason must also be submitted.

6. All screening data will be entered into a Wang computer by the secretarial coordinator in the Nutritional Assessment Center.

7. Output data will be graphically depicted on a Screening Nutrition Profile (Fig. 2) and interpreted by a clinical dietitian.

   Comprehensive nutritional assessment will be recommended for all patients with one or more of the following results:

   a. Weight for height: <80 percent of ideal weight.*
   b. History of unintentional weight loss: >10 lb or >5 percent of usual weight.
   c. Triceps skinfold: <80 percent of standard.**
   d. Arm muscle circumference: <80 percent of standard.**
   e. Serum albumin concentration: <3.5 g/dl.
   f. Total lymphocyte count: <1500 cells/mm^3.
   g. History of nausea, vomiting, diarrhea, dysphagia, abdominal pain or other gastrointestinal complaints that interfere with nutrient intake or absorption.

8. The nutrition technician will submit the completed Screening Nutrition Profile and recommendations to the progress notes of the medical record. Initial comprehensive nutritional assessment will be initiated within 12 hours after the order is received from the attending or resident physician.

REPORTING AND RECORDING

1. The nutrition technician will submit the Screening Nutrition Profile to the progress notes of the medical record.

2. When nutritional depletion is documented the clinical dietitian will submit a note to the progress notes of the medical record recommending indicated nutrition care.

---

* Ideal weights are derived from data reported in the Health and Nutritional Examination Survey I.[1]

** 50th percentile derived from data sets reported in the Health and Nutritional Examination Survey I.[2]

SCREENING NUTRITION PROFILE
HERMANN HOSPITAL/THE UNIVERSITY HOSPITAL

Addressograph

Name: _____ Room No.: _____ Physician: _____

Diagnosis: _____

	20	40	60	80	100	120	
Weight _____ Kg						%	Ideal weight

	20	40	60	80	100	120	
Usual Wt.: _____ Kg						%	Usual weight

	-15	-10	-5	0	+5	+10	
Wt. Change: _____ Kg						%	Weight change

	20	40	60	80	100	120	
Skinfold: _____ mm							Skinfold/ % STD

	20	40	60	80	100	120	
Arm muscle circ: _____ cm							Arm muscle circ/ % STD

	2.5	3.0	3.5	4.0	4.5	5.0	
Albumin: _____ g/dl							Albumin

	500	1000	1500	2000	2500	3000	
TLC: cells/ _____ mm³							Total Lymphocyte Count

Interpretation: _____

_____

_____

_____

Recommendation: _____

_____

_____

_____ R.D.

_____ M.D.

Figure 2. Screening Nutrition Profile. The Screening Nutrition Profile is submitted to the medical record to summarize data collected soon after admission to the hospital.

PATIENT TEACHING

1. Inform patient of purpose of triceps skinfold and arm circumference measurements.
2. Inform patient that interview is useful for planning subsequent nutritional care.

REFERENCES

1. National Center for Health Statistics. Weight by Height and Age of Adults 1-74 Years, 1971-1974. Advance Data 14, 1977.
2. Frisancho, A.R.: New norms of upper limb fat and muscle areas for assessment of nutritional status. Am. J. Clin. Nutr. 34:2540, 1981.

B. Procedure for Comprehensive Nutritional Assessment

PURPOSE

The purposes of the procedure for comprehensive nutritional assessment are:

1. To identify patients with marginal or overt nutritional depletion and to alert the health care team to the malnourished state.
2. To classify the type and degree of malnutrition and identify etiology.
3. To provide guidelines for planning nutrition care.
4. To evaluate response to nutrition therapy at designated intervals.

GENERAL INFORMATION

1. Indications for comprehensive nutritional assessment include the following as detected by screening nutritional assessment at admission to the hospital:
   a. Weight for height: <80 percent ideal weight.
   b. History of unintentional weight loss: >10 lb or >5 percent of usual weight.
   c. Triceps skinfold: <80 percent of standard.**
   d. Arm muscle circumference: <80 percent of standard.**
   e. Serum albumin concentration: <3.5 g/dl.
   f. Total lymphocyte count: <1500 cells/mm^3.
   g. History of nausea, vomiting, diarrhea, dysphagia or other gastrointestinal complaints which interfere with nutrient intake or absorption (see Section II-A).
2. All patients with diagnoses of multiple trauma and/or burns greater than 10 percent of total body surface will automatically be assessed since these hypermetabolic states are associated with nutritional depletion as a result of stress and increased energy and nutrient

* Ideal weights are derived from data reported in the Health and Nutritional Evaluation Survey I.[1]
** Standards derived from 50th percentile of data reported in the Health and Nutritional Examination Survey I.[2]

requirements. In these cases, comprehensive nutritional assessment will be initiated on the fifth postinjury day or following the resolution of fluid and electrolyte imbalances which may complicate interpretation of data.

3. Potential candidates for enteral and/or parenteral nutrition support will be assessed prior to the initiation of nutritional therapy.

4. Nutritional assessment must be ordered by the resident or attending physician in the physician's orders of the medical record. Preoperative nutritional assessment must be ordered as such to facilitate the most rapid communication of results and prevent delay of impending surgery.

5. The Nutritional Assessment General Orders must be signed by the resident or attending physician prior to initiation of data collection. The use of this form eliminates the need to reorder Nutritional Assessment at 10-day serial intervals.

6. Nutrition technicians, clinical dietitians, staff nurses, hyperalimentation nurses, and laboratory technicians from respective departments are involved in nutritional assessment data collection and comprise the multidisciplinary nutrition team.

7. All data collected for comprehensive nutritional assessment purposes will be delivered to the Nutritional Assessment Center, assimilated and interpreted by a clinical dietitian and physician.

8. The completed Nutritional Profile and Data Summary will be submitted to the progress notes of the medical record within 72 hours after data collection is initiated.

9. When nutritional depletion is documented on the initial profile, a nutrition care plan will be recommended in the progress notes of the medical record by the clinical dietitian. Nutritional Assessment will continue serially until all nutritional indices are within normal limits.

EQUIPMENT

Equipment is listed under each procedure for data collection (see Sections II-C thru II-P).

PROCEDURE

1. Nutritional Assessment is ordered by the attending physician or resident on the Physician's Orders in the medical record.

2. The initial order for nutritional assessment is communicated to the Department of Dietetics and Nutrition in the same manner that diet orders are communicated.

3. Within 12 hours after receiving the initial order, a nutritional technician from the Nutritional Assessment Program will sign and submit the Nutritional Assessment General Orders (Fig. 3) to the Physician's Orders section of the medical record.

4. Within 12 hours after receiving the initial order for nutritional assessment, the nutrition technician will initiate data collection as follows:

   a. Record the patient's height on the Profile Data Record (Fig. 4) (see Section II-C).

PHYSICIAN'S ORDERS

HERMANN HOSPITAL / THE UNIVERSITY HOSPITAL

ALLERGIES_____

"Authorization is hereby given to dispense
the Generic or Chemical equivalent unless
otherwise indicated by the words —
NO SUBSTITUTE"

ORDERED		ORDERS
DATE	TIME	

NUTRITIONAL ASSESSMENT GENERAL ORDERS

I. Notify IVH Nurse to:

1. Apply skin test antigens.
   Inject 0.1 ml of each antigen into dermis of volar aspect of forearm.

Mumps	Trichophytin PPD (intermediate strength)
Candida	SK-SD (streptokinase-streptodornase)

2. Read response at 24 and 48 hours.
3. Repeat entire protocol every ten days.

II. Notify Nursing Staff to:
   1. Record 24 hour intake of food and fluids from 7:00 a.m. to 7:00 a.m. daily.

   a. Include all enteral (food and fluid) and parenteral (IV and IVH) intake on record form.
   b. Place menus from tray in Nutritional Assessment Envelope.

   2. Weight patient daily.
      a. Weigh patient before breakfast in hospital gown only.

   b. Record daily weights with nutrient intakes on form entitled
      "Nutrient Intake and Weight Record."

   3. Collect 24 hour urine from 7:00 a.m. to 7:00 a.m. on _____.

III. Notify Dietetics Department to:

   1. Complete the initial patient interview.
   2. Calculate daily nutrient intakes from enteral and parenteral sources.

   3. Measure anthropometrics.
      Height

      Triceps skinfold
      Mid-arm circumference

   4. Order laboratory testing.

      Serum albumin
      Serum transferrin

      Prealbumin
      Retinol-binding protein
      Serum osmolarity

      WBC with differential and lymphocyte count
      24 hour urine for urea nitrogen and creatinine

   5. Repeat anthropometric measurements (excluding height) and laboratory testing
      every 10 days.

   6. Calculate average energy and nutrient intakes every 10 days.

_____ M.D.

Transcribed by: _____

Figure 3. Nutritional Assessment General Order Set. The chart approved standard order set for nutritional assessment permits organized communication of tests and procedures necessary for initial and serial assessments.

b. Weigh the patient and record the weight on the Profile Data Record. If a bed scale is required to weigh the patient, the nutrition technician will notify the primary nurse to weigh the patient (see Section II-D or II-E).

c. Measure arm circumference and triceps skinfold three times and record average measurements on the Profile Data Record (see Section II-F or II-G).

d. Initiate daily nutrient intake and explain procedures for accu-

NUTRITIONAL ASSESSMENT PROFILE DATA RECORD
HERMANN HOSPITAL/*The University Hospital*

DEMOGRAPHIC DATA

Name _____

Physician _____

Technician _____

Dietitian _____

Room No. _____ Assessment No. _____

Hospital No. _____ Assessment Date _____

Sex _____ Age _____

HOSPITAL COURSE

Diagnosis _____

Nutrition Prescription _____

Sepsis _____

Surgical Procedures/Dates _____

_____

Complications _____

ANTHROPOMETRIC DATA

Height ——————— (in.)

Present Wt. ——————— (lb.)

Usual Wt. ——————— (lb.)

Date(MMDDYY) ———————

Admission Wt. ——————— (lb.)

Date (MMDDYY) ———————

Tricaps Skinfold ——————— (mm)

Arm Circumference ——————— (cm)

Biceps Skinfold ——————— (mm)

Subscapular Skinfold ——————— (mm)

Supra-iliac Skinfold ——————— (mm)

SKIN TEST DATA

Trychophytin ——————— (mm induration - 48 hr.)

Candica ——————— (mm induration - 48 hr.)

Mumps ——————— (mm induration - 48 hr.)

Intermediate PPD ——————— (mm induration - 48 hr.)

LABORATORY DATA

24 hr. Urine Creatinine ——————— (mg/dl)

Total Urine Volume ——————— (ml)

Serum Albumin ——————— (mg/dl)

Serum Transferrin ——————— (mg/dl)

Prealbumin ——————— (mg/dl)

Retinol Binding Protein ——————— (mg/dl)

Serum Osmolarity ——————— (mOsm/l)

Lymphocytes ——————— (percent)

White Blood Cells ——————— (cells/mm^3)

24 hr. Urine Urea Nitrogen ——————— (mg/dl)

NUTRIENT INTAKE DATA

Calorie Intake (24 hr. intake) ——————— (Kcal)

Protein Intake (24 hr. intake) ——————— (g)

Stress Code ———————
HH/752-02(10/80R)MR

Calorie Intake (10 day average) ——————— (Kcal)

Protein Intake (10 day average) ——————— (g)

Figure 4. Profile Data Record. All incoming data from team members is assimilated on the Profile Data Record.

rate record completion to the patient and primary nurse (see Section II-I).

e. Notify the primary nurse of orders for daily weights, 24-hour urine collection and nutrient intake records and review procedures to ensure accurate data collection. These orders will also be communicated through usual channels and implemented according to standard procedure (see Sections II-D, II-E, II-J and II-M).

f. Complete Nutritional Assessment Laboratory Requisitions for the following tests if they have not been ordered within the previous 24 hours:

> Serum albumin.
> Serum transferrin.
> Prealbumin.
> Retinol-binding protein.
> Serum osmolarity.
> White blood cell count.
> Differential for lymphocytes.
> 24-hour urine urea nitrogen.
> 24-hour urine creatinine.
> (See Section II-L).

g. Notify nutrition support nurses of orders for skin antigen testing.

5. Nutrition support nurses will check floor stock of skin test antigen solutions, notify pharmacy if additional solution is needed, prepare syringes for injections, and administer skin test antigens on the following day (see Sections II-N and II-O).

6. The nutrition support nurse will read skin test reactions 24 and 48 hours following injection and communicate results to the Nutritional Assessment Center (see Section II-P).

7. Within 72 hours after receiving the order for Nutritional Assessment, a clinical dietitian will review the patient's medical record and complete the direct patient interview.

8. A nutrition technician will collect Food and Fluid Intake Records and calculate daily energy and nutrient intakes (see Section II-K).

9. All initial data from nutrition technicians, nurses, and laboratory technicians will be delivered to the Nutritional Assessment Center and transcribed onto the Profile Data Record.

10. The secretarial coordinator will type all data into the computer and complete the Nutritional Profiles (Fig. 5) for review.

11. A clinical dietitian specialist and physician will review and interpret the Nutritional Profile and determine the nutrition diagnosis. The probable etiology of malnutrition including effects of surgical procedures, medications and complications will be noted in the interpretation. Suggestions for modifying the nutrition prescription will also be recorded (see Section III).

12. The signed and completed Nutritional Profile and Data Summary

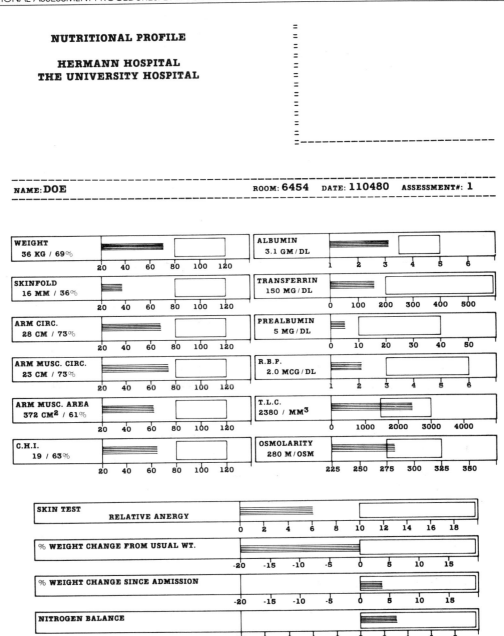

Figure 5. Nutritional Profile. A clinical dietitian and physician review and interpret the completed Nutritional Profile to determine the nutritional diagnosis. The probable etiology of malnutrition including effects of medications, surgical procedures and stress are noted in the interpretation. Recommendations for modifying nutritional therapy are also cited.

NUTRITIONAL PROFILE - DATA SUMMARY
HERMANN HOSPITAL/THE UNIVERSITY HOSPITAL

Name ....:Test Patient
Date ....:110480
Assessment # ....: 1

Nutritional : High Protein/High Calorie Diet
Support ......:
Diagnosis . : Gun Shot Wound to Abdomen
Surgery .....:11/01/80 Exploratory Lap
Complications ....: No

ANTHROPOMETRIC ASSESSMENT

Height	: 152 cm	Creatinine	: 19 mg
Weight	: 36 kg	Ideal Creatinine	: 927 mg
Ideal Weight	: 52 kg	Urine Volume	: 3052 ml
Weight/Ideal	: 69%	CHI/STD	: 63%
Admission Weight	: 35kg	Usual Weight	: 49 kg
Admission Date	: 101180	Usual Date	: 050280
Weight Change	: 3%	Weight Change	- 27%
Time Elapsed	: 3 wk	Time Elapsed	: 27 wk
Triceps Skinfold	: 6 mm	Skinfold/STD	: 36%
Arm Circumference	: 18.6 cm	Arm Circumference/STD	: 65%
Arm Muscle Circumference	: 17 cm	Arm Muscle Circ./STD	: 73%
Arm Muscle Area	: 229 cm^2	Arm Muscle Area/STD	: 61%

LABORATORY ASSESSMENT   :   SKIN ANTIGEN TESTING

Serum Albumin	: 3.1 gm/dl	Dermatophytin	: 4 mm
Serum Transferrin	: 150 mg/dl	Candida	: 0 mm
Retinol Binding Protein	: 4 mcg/dl	Varidase	: 0 mm
Prealbumin	: 10 mg/dl	Mumps	: 4 mm
Total Lymphocyte Count	: 2380 /mm^3	PPD	: 0 mm
Serum Osmoarlity	: 280 mOsm/1	Result	: Relative Anergy

INTAKE ASSESSMENT

Calorie Intake	: 2771 kcal	Basal Energy Expenditure	: 1051 kcal
Protein Intake	: 68 gms	Nitrogen Balance	: 3 gm
Calorie Intake (Average)	: 2519 kcal	Calorie Requirement	: 1577 kcal
Protein Intake (Average)	: 79 gms	Protein Requirement	: 66 gms

Figure 6. Nutritional Profile—Data Summary. The Nutritional Profile—Data Summary lists all assimilated data and is submitted to the medical record following each assessment.

(Fig. 6) will be submitted to the medical record by the nutrition technician within 72 hours after the initial order is received.

13. The clinical dietitian will submit a nutrition note to the progress notes of the medical record summarizing pertinent nutrition information from the review of the medical record, the patient's interview and the Nutrition Profile. Calculated nutrient requirements and recommendations for nutrition care will also be submitted (see Section III).

14. If nutritional depletion is documented, nutritional assessment will continue serially. The secretarial coordinator will plan, organize and communicate subsequent data collection as follows:

Weight	Daily
Energy and nutrient intakes	Daily
Skinfold and arm circumference measurements	Every 10 days
24-hour urine collection	Every 10 days
Laboratory testing	Every 10 days
Skin antigen testing	Every 10 days
Average energy and nutrient intakes	Every 10 days

When surgery is scheduled on the nutritional assessment date, nutritional assessment will be postponed until two days postoperatively.

15. A complete Nutritional Profile and Data Summary will be generated every 10 days and submitted to the medical record every 12 days until nutritional assessment is discontinued.

16. Each patient will be interviewed twice weekly by a clinical dietitian while on nutritional assessment to ascertain acceptance and tolerance of therapy.

17. When indicated, the clinical dietitian will modify nutrition care plans and submit recommendations for diet prescriptions, supplemental feedings, tube feedings and/or intravenous hyperalimentation to the medical record.

18. Nutritional assessment will be discontinued when all indices are within normal limits.

RECORDING AND REPORTING

1. Energy and nutrient intakes and daily weights are recorded in the progress notes of the medical record daily by nutrition technicians.

2. Skin test administration and results are recorded in the progress notes of the medical records after each application by the nutrition support nurse.

3. A completed Nutrition Profile and Data Summary are submitted to the medical record within 72 hours after the initial order is received and every 12 days thereafter until nutritional assessment is discontinued.

4. A chart copy of all laboratory testing for nutritional assessment purposes is submitted to the laboratory section of the medical record by the laboratory technician.
5. A nutrition note will be recorded in the progress notes of the medical record summarizing pertinent nutrition data from the medical record, patient interviews and the Nutrition Profile by the clinical dietitian following each comprehensive assessment.

PATIENT TEACHING

1. The nutrition technician will explain the purpose of the nutritional assessment procedure to the patient.
2. The clinical dietitian will review pertinent nutritional assessment data with the patient and ensure that the patient understands the importance of nutritional assessment procedures.

REFERENCES

1. National Center for Health Statistics. Weight by Height and Age of Adults 1-74 Years; 1971-1974. Advance Data 14, 1977.
2. Frisancho, A.R.: New norms of upper limb fat and muscle areas for assessment of nutritional status. Am. J. Clin. Nutr. 34:2540, 1981.

C. Procedure for Measuring Stature Using a Balance Scale

The purposes of the procedure for measuring stature using a balance scale are:

1. To define a procedure for measurement of body height that is readily accessible on all patient floors.
2. To provide an index for comparison of body weight measurements with ideal weight for height standards.
3. To provide an index for comparison of creatinine excretion with published standards.

GENERAL INFORMATION

1. Height is routinely measured by a nutrition technician from the Nutritional Assessment Program as part of the screening nutritional assessment procedure.
2. Weight for height is the most commonly used indicator of nutritional status. Stature (standing height) is defined as the distance from the sole of the feet to the top of the head.
3. The creatinine/height index provides an estimate of skeletal muscle mass because urinary levels of creatinine are dependent principally upon the extent of skeletal muscle catabolism. The creatinine/height index compares 24-hour creatinine excretion of the patient with expected creatinine excretion of a normal adult of the same height. Accurate measurements of height are essential for data interpretation.
4. The patient must be measured without shoes since standards used for interpretation of weight for height data are based on heights without shoes.

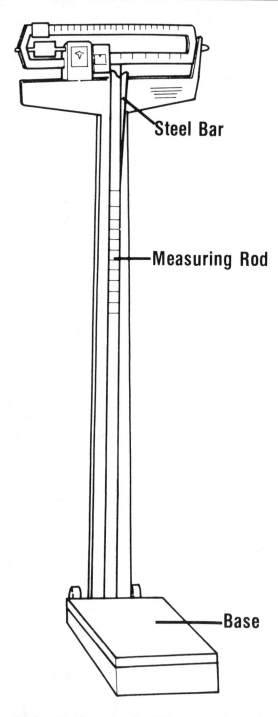

Figure 7. Balance Scale with Measuring Rod. The measuring rod and steel bar on the balance scale are used to measure stature.

5. The parts of the platform balance scale that are essential to measure height are (Fig. 7):

   a. Base: The patient stands in the center of the base when height is measured.

   b. Measuring rod: The measuring rod is adjustable and contains the measurement scale which is calibrated in inches. The actual height in inches is read at the base of the adjustable rod to the nearest 1/4 inch.

   c. Steel bar: The steel bar extends vertically from the measuring rod and is lowered over the patient's head.

EQUIPMENT

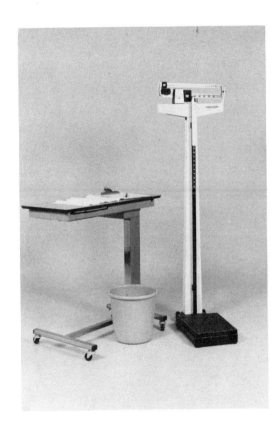

- Platform balance scale with measuring rod
- Paper towel
- Pen or pencil
- Screening Nutritional Assessment Data Card

PROCEDURE

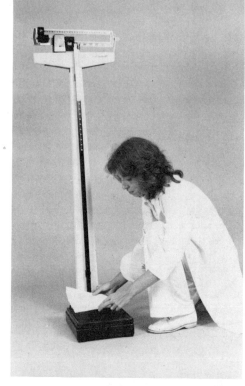

1. Place a paper towel on the center of the scale base for cleanliness and as protection from possible contamination.

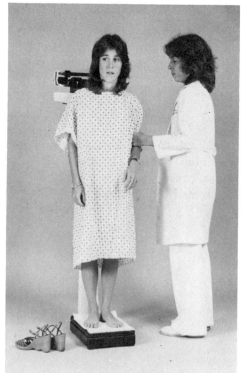

2. Instruct the patient to remove shoes and step onto the paper towel with his or her back to the measuring rod.

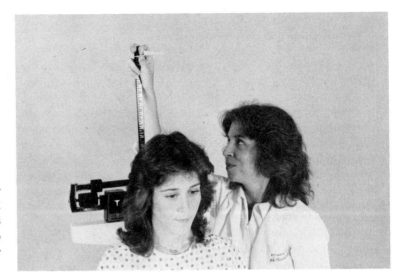

3. Raise the measuring rod until it is approximately six inches above the patient's head and raise the steel bar so that it is extended vertically over the patient's head.

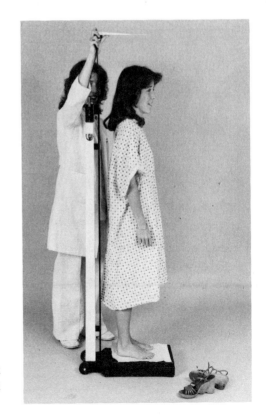

4. Instruct the patient to stand erect so that the line of sight is horizontal and the heels and scapulae are aligned with the measuring rod.

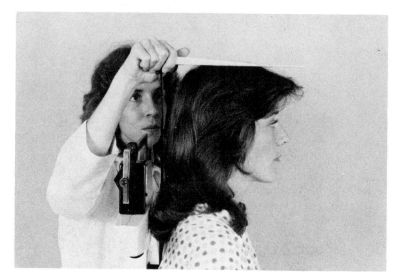

5. Lower the steel bar until it just makes contact with the patient's scalp. Instruct the patient to step down and put on his or her shoes.

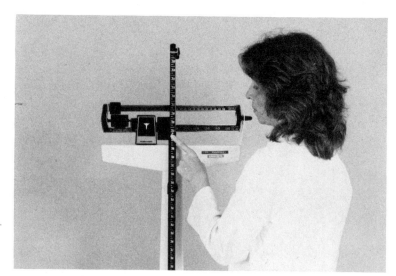

6. Read the height to the nearest 1/4 inch at the base of the adjustable measuring rod. Record this reading.

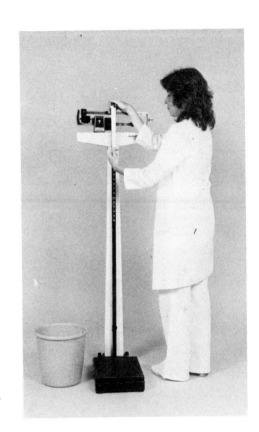

7. Return the bar and measuring rod to the original position. Discard the paper towel in the waste container.

REPORTING AND RECORDING

1. Record the patient's height in inches on the Screening Nutritional Assessment Data Card.
2. Indicate a verbal height if the patient is unable to be measured.
3. Return the complete Screening Nutritional Assessment Data Card to the Nutritional Assessment Center.

REFERENCE

1. Bonewit, K.: The physical examination, in Clinical Procedures for Medical Assistants. Philadelphia: W.B. Saunders, 1979, p. 59.

D. Procedure for Measuring Weight Using a Platform Balance Scale _____

The purposes of the procedure for measuring weights using a platform balance scale are:

1. To provide an indication of nutritional status and fluid balance.
2. To provide objective guidelines for monitoring the effectiveness of nutritional therapy and altering subsequent care plans.

GENERAL INFORMATION

1. Body weight is the most commonly used indicator of nutritional status and fluid balance and is an important component of screening and comprehensive nutritional assessment procedures.
2. Since weight can vary throughout the day, accurate daily weights must be taken at the same time every day. To ensure accurate and comparable weight recordings, the weight is taken in the morning after the patient has voided and before he has eaten.
3. The patient must wear the same amount of clothing (preferably the hospital gown only) and no shoes during each weighing.
4. The same scale must be used every day.
5. Daily weights are the responsibility of the staff nurse on the 11:00 P.M. to 7:00 A.M. shift.
6. When a weight gain greater than one pound per 24 hours is noted, the patient is retaining some excessive fluid, and shortness of breath and/or ankle edema should be observed and reported if noted.
7. There are six essential parts of the balance scale (Fig. 8):

    a. Base: The patient stands erect in the center of the base.
    b. Trig-loop: The trig-loop surrounds the beam pointer and restricts its movement.

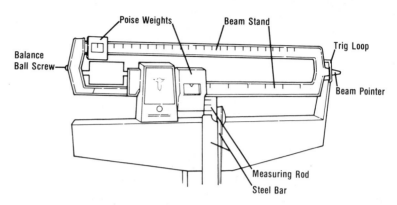

Figure 8. Platform Balance Scale. The platform balance scale is used to weigh ambulatory patients in the upright position.

   c. Beam pointer: The beam pointer should float gently up and
      down without touching the trig-loop when the scale is balanced.
   d. Balance ball screw: The balance ball screw is used to balance
      the scale. If the beam pointer stabilizes below the center of the
      trig-loop, the balance ball screw is turned clockwise until the
      beam is in balance. If the beam pointer stabilizes above the
      center line of the trig-loop, the balance ball screw is turned
      counterclockwise until the beam is in balance.
   e. Poise weight(s):   When weighing the patient, the upper and
      lower poise weights are moved to the right, towards the beam
      pointer, until the beam pointer floats gently up and down with-
      out touching either the top or bottom of the trig-loop.
   f. Beam stand(s):   The upper beam stand is calibrated in 1/4-
      pound increments, and the lower beam stand is calibrated in
      50-pound increments. The lower poise weight rests on the "V"
      shaped bearings on the beam stand.

8. The platform balance scale must be tested every six months and
   serviced by a qualified scale mechanic if necessary.

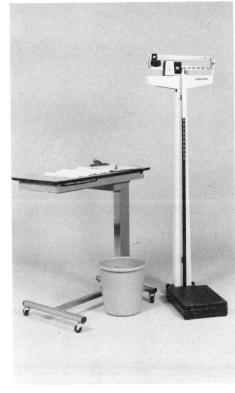

EQUIPMENT

- Platform balance scale
- Pen or pencil
- Nurse's notes
- Paper towel

PROCEDURE

1. Balance the scale prior to weighing in order to insure accuracy of the weight measurement.

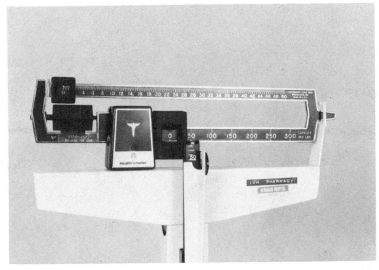

a. When the scale is balanced, the beam pointer should float gently up and down and not touch either the top or bottom of the trig-loop, when both poise weights are placed on "0."

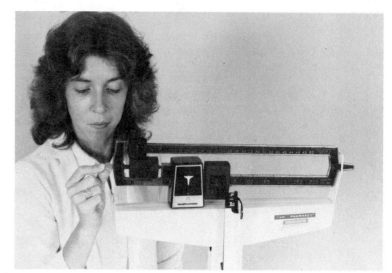

b. If the beam pointer touches the bottom or stabilizes below the center line of the trig-loop, the balance ball screw is turned clockwise using a penny until the beam pointer is in balance.

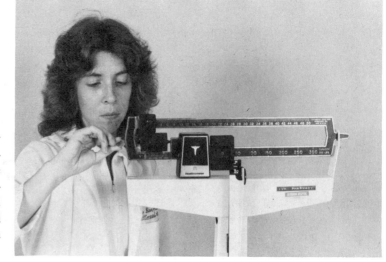

c. If the beam pointer touches the top or stabilizes above the center line of the trig-loop, the balance ball screw is turned counterclockwise until the beam pointer is in balance.

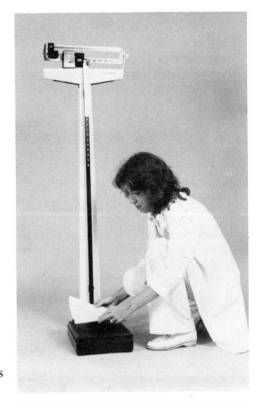

2. Place a paper towel on the base for cleanliness and as protection from possible contamination.

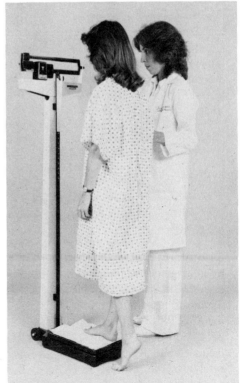

3. Assist the patient with removal of shoes and all clothing except hospital gown and assist onto the scale. Instruct subject to stand erect in the center of the scale.

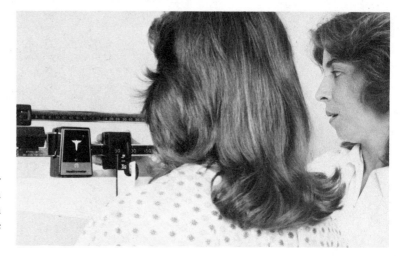

4. Balance the scale by positioning the lower poise weight in the "V" shaped bearing on the beam stand closest to the patient's usual weight.

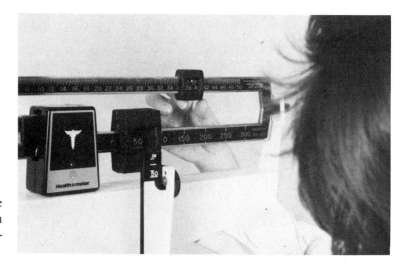

5. Then, move the upper poise weight towards the beam pointer until the scale is balanced.

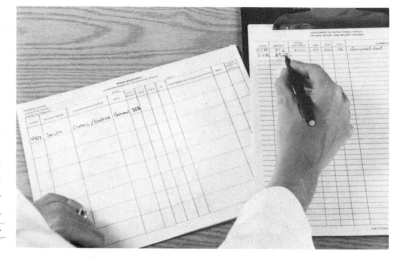

6. Calculate the patient's weight by adding the reading indicated by the poise weight on the lower beam stand to the reading indicated by the poise weight on the upper beam stand. Record accurately to the nearest 1/4 pound.

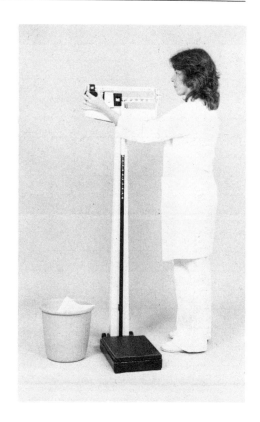

7. Return poise weights to the "0" position. Discard the paper towel in the waste container.

REPORTING AND RECORDING

1. Record reading in the "Nurse's Notes."
2. When daily weights are ordered for Nutritional Assessment, weight must also be recorded on the form entitled "Calorie Intake and Weight Record" (Fig. 9).

REFERENCES

1. Bonewit, K.: Procedure for measuring weight, in Clinical Procedures for Medical Assistants. Philadelphia: W.B. Saunders, 1979, p. 59.
2. Broadwell, L. and Milutinovic, B.: Selected nursing measures, in Medical Surgical Nursing Procedures. Albany, N.Y.: Dalmar Publishers, 1979, p. 98.

CALORIE INTAKE AND WEIGHT RECORD

DATE	WEIGHT	TOTAL CALORIES	CHO	PRO	FAT	COMMENTS

HH/803-35(10/77)

DIETITIAN _____

Figure 9. Calorie Intake and Weight Record. Serial daily weights are recorded on this form with daily energy and nutrient intakes to provide a basis for evaluating changes in recorded weights.

52

E. Procedure for Measuring Weight Using a Bed Scale

The purposes of the procedure for measuring weights using a bed scale are:

1. To measure accurately body weight and daily fluctuations in weight for those patients who cannot assume the upright position for weighing on a platform balance scale.
2. To provide an indication of nutritional status and fluid balance.
3. To provide objective guidelines for monitoring the effectiveness of nutrition therapy and altering subsequent care plans.

1. Body weight is the most commonly used indicator of nutritional status and fluid balance and is an important component of screening and comprehensive nutritional assessment procedures.
2. Since weight can vary throughout the day, accurate daily weights must be taken at the same time every day. To ensure accurate and comparable weight recordings, the weight is taken in the morning after the patient has voided and before he has eaten.
3. The patient must wear the same amount of clothing (preferably the hospital gown only) and no shoes during each weighing.
4. The same scale must be used every day.
5. Daily weights are the responsibility of the staff nurse on the 11:00 P.M. to 7:00 A.M. shift.
6. When weight gain greater than one pound per 24 hours is noted, the patient is retaining some excessive fluid and shortness of breath and/or ankle edema should be noted if observed.
7. Although many bed scales are available, this procedure is defined for use of the Scale-Tronix 2001 Lift Bed scale since this scale is most commonly used in this hospital.
   The Scale-Tronix 2001 lift bed scale is a medical scale exclusively

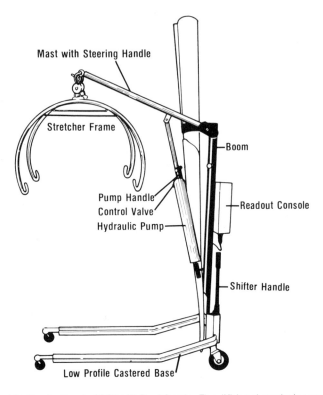

Mast with Steering Handle

Stretcher Frame

Boom

Pump Handle
Control Valve
Hydraulic Pump

Readout Console

Shifter Handle

Low Profile Castered Base

Figure 10. Scale-Tronix 2001 Lift Bed Scale. The lift bed scale is used to weigh those patients who cannot assume the upright position for weighing on a platform balance scale. Disposable stretchers are available to minimize the possibility of infection for those patients in protective isolation.

designed for weighing patients who cannot stand on the balance scale. It is composed of nine major mechanical parts identified as follows (Fig. 10):

  a. Low profile castered base: The tubular steel base with full swivel casters supports the scale structure. The base legs can be spread apart for greater stability and safety during weighing. The base also contains a shelf for storing the stretcher when not in use.

  b. Shifter handle: This handle spreads and locks the legs of the base to the open position. It also locks the legs in the closed position to allow for easier movement through doorways.

  c. Boom: This tubular steel structure supports the stretcher over the bed.

  d. Mast with steering handle: The tubular steel mast supports the boom and readout console. A spring clip is attached to the top of the mast to hold the stretcher for storage.

e. Stretcher frame: This tubular steel structure holds the stretcher fabric that supports the patient. The stretcher frame will also hold disposable stretchers which can be purchased specifically for weighing the patient in protective isolation. The stretcher frame contains weighing load sensors which measure the patient's weight.

f,g,h. Hydraulic pump, pump handle and control valve: The sealed pump with handle controls lifting of the patient slightly out of bed. The control valve gently lowers the patient back to bed.

i. Readout console: This electronic instrument displays the patient's weight directly in pounds. It contains rechargeable batteries.

8. The scale is intended for use as a scale only and should never be used to transport patients.

9. The patient must never be moved away from the bed or the bed must never be moved away from the scale while the patient is suspended on the scale.

10. The patient must never be left unattended while on the scale.

11. The lift scale must be tested once every six months and serviced, if necessary, by a qualified scale mechanic.

EQUIPMENT

- Scale-Tronix 2001 lift bed scale with stretcher
- Pen or pencil
- Nurse's notes
- Calorie intake and weight record

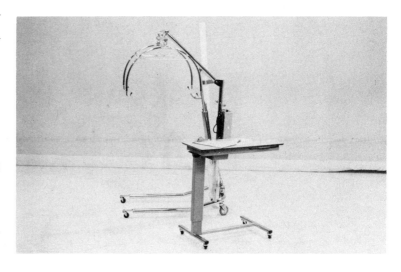

PROCEDURE

1. Determine the empty weight of the stretcher as follows:

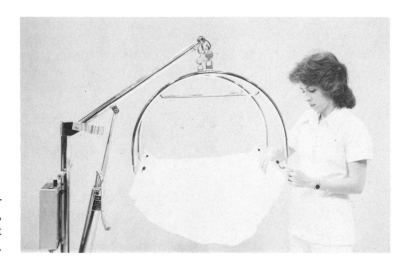

a. Attach the empty stretcher to the frame hooks, checking to assure that it is not touching anything.

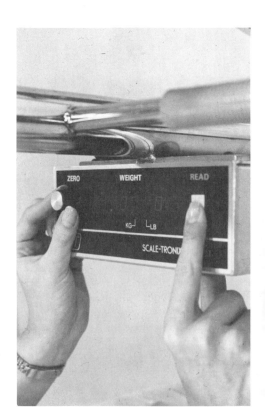

b. Press the "read" button on the readout console and hold it down. Adjust the scale to read 00.0 by turning the "zero" knob on the readout console. Remove the stretcher fabric and bars from frame hooks.

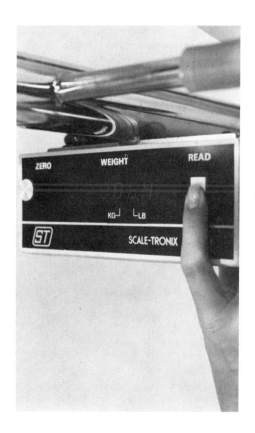

c. Press "read" button and note reading after three seconds. Note and record this number, it is the actual weight of the stretcher fabric and bars.

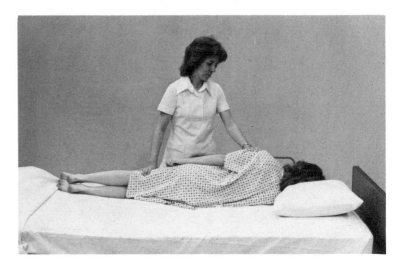

2. Turn the patient on his side (or have him turn) to make room for the stretcher fabric to be spread over the mattress.

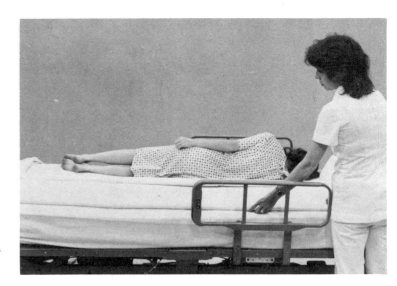

3. Place the stretcher fabric (with bars inserted) over the mattress and position the patient so that the heels are a few inches over one end of the fabric.

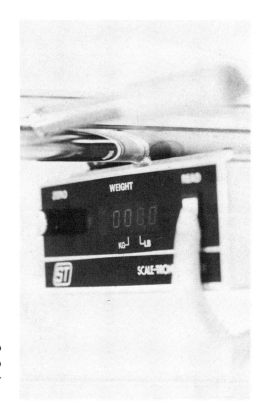

4. Before attaching the scale, press the "read" button to check the scale setting and adjust the "zero" knob to subtract the previously obtained empty stretcher weight.

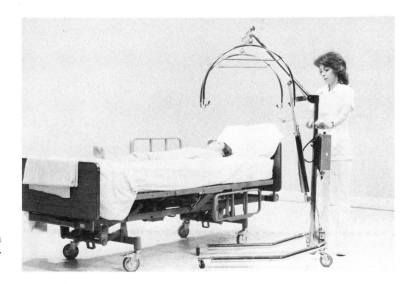

5. Move the scale into position next to bed with stretcher frame over patient.

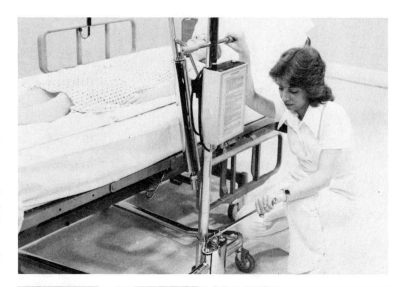

6. To spread the legs of the scale base, first grasp the shifter handle in one hand and place the opposite hand on the steering handle of the mast for balance. Then rotate the shifter handle 45 degrees to the right, and pull forward in a complete half circle.

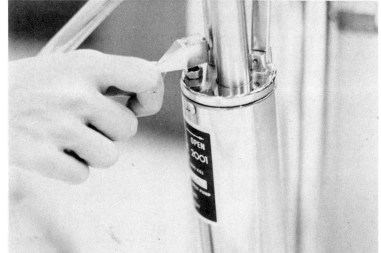

7. Open the control valve to lower gently the stretcher frame over the patient.

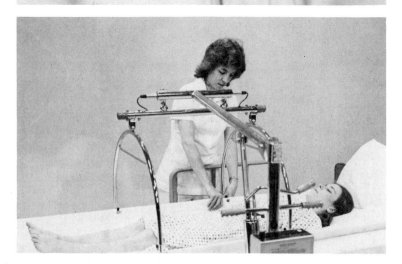

8. Attach the stretcher bars to all four hooks in the frame.

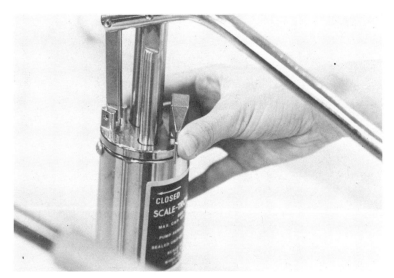

9. Close the control valve.

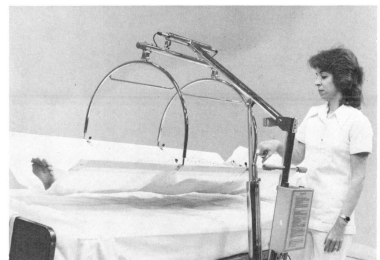

10. Gently operate the pump to lift the patient two inches off the bed.

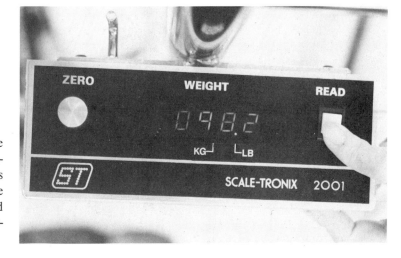

11. After checking to assure that the patient and stretcher are hanging freely, press the "read" button and note the weight in pounds and kilograms after three seconds.

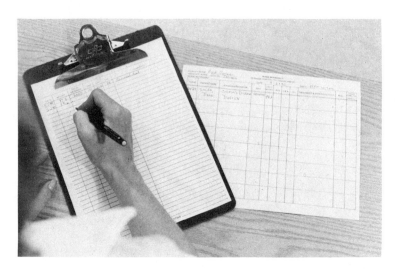

12. Record this reading.

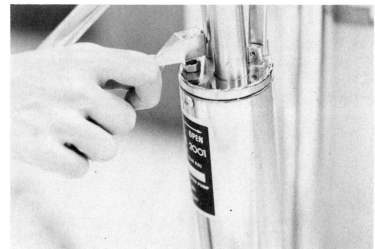

13. Open the control valve to lower slowly the patient back into bed.

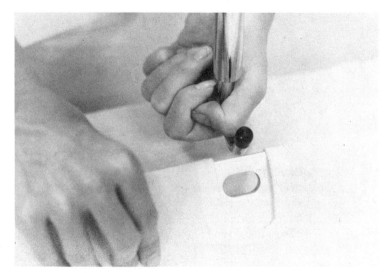

14. Disconnect the stretcher frame from stretcher bars.

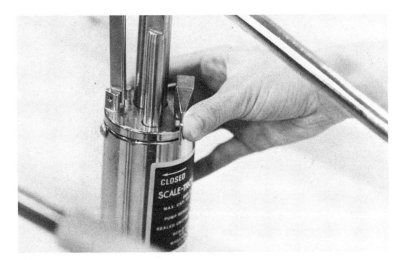

15. Close the control valve to raise stretcher frame.

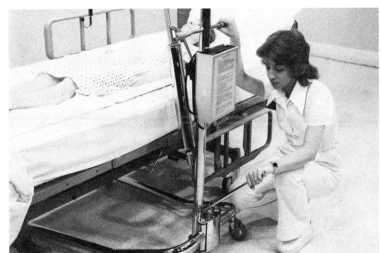

16. Close the base legs with the shifter handle and move the scale away from the bed side.

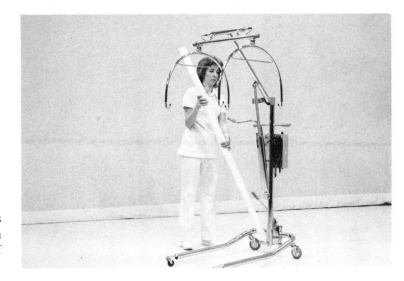

17. Roll up the stretcher bars and fabric and place them on the shelf at the base of the scale.

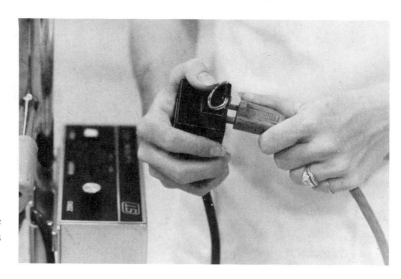

18. Plug in the scale to charge
the batteries at all times
when not in use.

**REPORTING AND
RECORDING**

1. Record reading in the "Nurse's Notes."
2. When daily weights are ordered for nutritional assessment purposes weights must also be recorded on the form entitled "Calorie Intake and Weight Record" (see Fig. 9).

REFERENCE

1. Scale-Tronix 2001 Bed Scale, Instruction and Service Manual.

F. Procedure for Measuring
Arm Circumference and Triceps Skinfold
in the Standard Position _____

The purposes of the procedure for measuring arm circumference and skinfolds in the standard position are:

1. To assess the status of body fat and somatic protein (skeletal muscle) stores.
2. To identify those patients who are nutritionally at risk.
3. To evaluate patient response to nutrition therapy.

1. The following anthropometric measurements are routinely included in the screening and comprehensive nutritional assessment procedures:
   a. Location of upper arm midpoint.
   b. Midupper arm circumference.
   c. Triceps skinfold.
2. Adipose tissue, the primary caloric reserve of the body, is assessed by measuring the triceps skinfold, which includes the subcutaneous fat layer.
3. The arm muscle circumference and arm muscle area are calculated from triceps skinfold and arm circumference measurements. These calculations indicate the status of somatic protein stores.
4. All anthropometric measurements are performed by nutrition technicians from the Department of Dietetics, Nutritional Assessment Program. To ensure the most accurate and comprehensive measurements, all initial and serial measurements on a given patient will be performed by the same technician when possible.
5. All constricting clothes and garments must be removed prior to measurement.
6. Measurements are taken with the patient standing erect when possible. If the patient is unable to stand or sit upright, arm

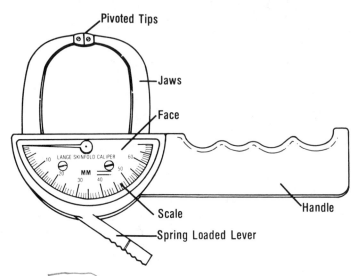

Figure 11. Lange® Skinfold Caliper. The Lange skinfold caliper is specifically designed for simple accurate measurement of skinfolds.

measurements may be taken in the supine position as directed in the Section II-G.

7. Arm measurements should be taken on the right side of the body when possible since standards for comparison are based on right arm measurements.

8. Careful adherence to precise procedure and technique is essential to ensure accuracy of measurement. Any deviation from these guidelines and procedures must be recorded with the measurement.

9. All anthropometric measurements are repeated serially at 10-day intervals to assess changes in nutritional status and response to therapy.

10. The Lange® skinfold caliper, manufactured by Cambridge Scientific Industries, Cambridge, Maryland, is specifically designed for simple accurate measurement of skinfolds. The Lange Caliper® is comprised of the following parts (Fig. 11):

  a. Handle: The handle of the Lange caliper provides a molded grip for ease of handling.

  b. Spring loaded lever: The spring loaded lever provides a constant standard pressure of 10 g/sq mm over the entire operating range. This lever is depressed with the thumb of the right hand to open the caliper jaws.

  c. Caliper jaws: The caliper jaws are of sturdy lightweight construction and are opened by depressing the spring loaded lever.

  d. Pivoted tips: The pivoted tips are located at the opening of each caliper jaw and adjust automatically for parallel measurement of skinfolds. All critical pivot points utilize low fric-

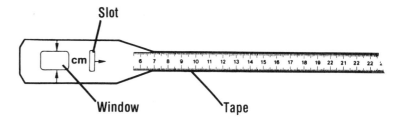

Figure 12. Insertion tape. Midupper arm circumference can be measured easily with an insertion tape which eliminates some of the technical errors inherent with the use of standard tapes.

tion bearings to maintain accurate tip pressure at the jaw openings and assure patient comfort.

  e. Face and scale: The face is approximately 30 mm and contains the scale which permits reading up to 70 mm accurate to ±1 mm.

11. The arm circumference is most accurately measured using an Insertion Tape®. This tape offers improved control and alignment and eliminates some of the technical errors inherent with the use of standard tapes. The insertion tape consists of the following basic parts (Fig. 12):

  a. Tape: The actual tape contains the measuring scale which is calibrated in centimeters.

  b. Slot: The distal end of the tape is threaded through the slot in the origin to tighten the tape around the arm.

  c. Window: The actual measurement is read through the window at the origin of the tape. Vertical pointed arrows indicate the exact measurement.

EQUIPMENT

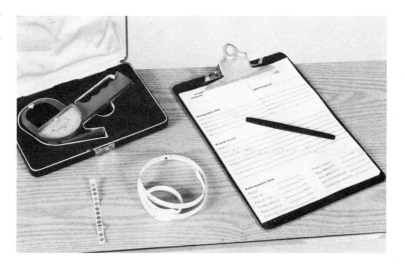

- Lange skinfold caliper with constant pressure of 10 g/sq mm
- Insertion tape
- Pen or pencil
- Nutritional Assessment Data Card or Record
- Adhesive labels

PROCEDURE

Location of the upper arm midpoint:

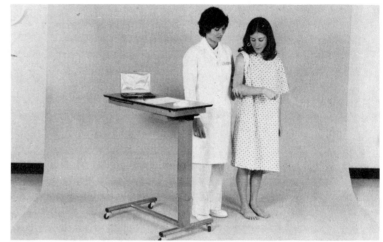

1. Instruct the patient to stand erect, bend the right arm at a 90° angle from the elbow and make a fist.

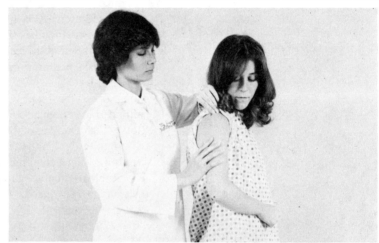

2. Locate the tip of the olecranon process of the ulna and the acromial process of the scapula by palpation and mark these sites with adhesive labels while palpating (Fig. 13).

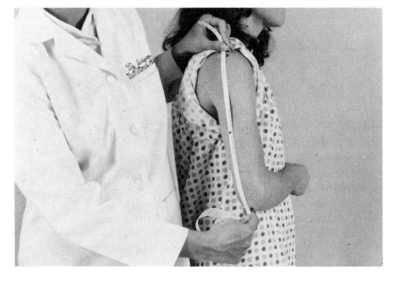

3. Place the zero inch mark of the insertion tape against the marked tip of the acromial process and run the tape down the posterior side of the upper arm to the marked tip of the olecranon process.

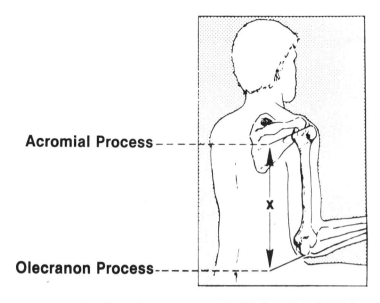

Acromial Process

Olecranon Process

Figure 13. Identification of upper arm midpoint. The midpoint of the upper arm is located midway between the tip of the olecranon process of the ulna and the acromial process of the scapula.

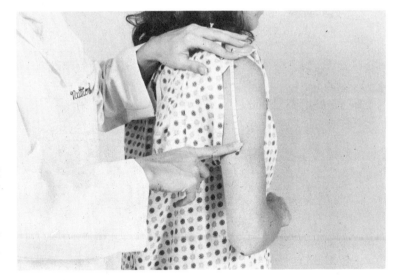

4. Loop the tape in half, joining the two measured ends at the tip of the acromial process. Mark the midpoint at the end of the loop directly *in line* with the olecranon process using an adhesive label.

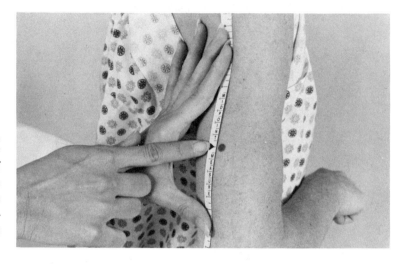

5. When using the Inser-tape*, adjust the tape vertically along the posterior aspect of the upper arm until the same number appears at the marked acromial and olecranon processes. "Zero" is the midpoint.

Measurement of mid-upper arm circumference:

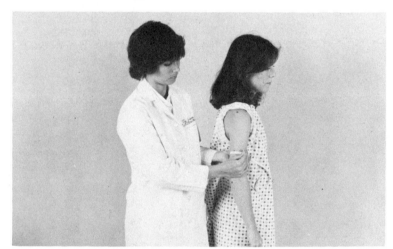

1. Measure the right arm as it hangs freely.

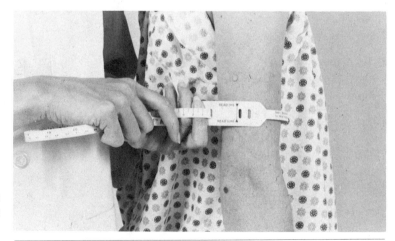

2. Thread the distal end of the insertion tape through the slot in the proximal end.

---

* Inser-tape®, Ross Laboratories, Columbus, Ohio.

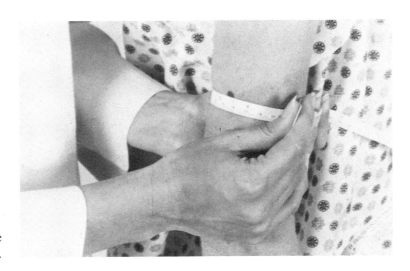

3. Align the upper edge of the tape with the midpoint mark.

4. Tighten the tape until it is in contact with the skin without constricting it. Read the arm circumference through the window at the origin of the tape to the nearest 0.1 cm.

5. Record the measurement.

Measurement of triceps skinfold:

1. Measure the right arm as it hangs freely at the side. Pick up a lengthwise, vertical, double-fold of skin and fat about 1 cm above the midpoint mark, between the thumb and the forefinger of the left hand. The skinfold should be directly in line with the point of the olecranon process. Pull the fold cleanly away from the underlying muscle. Have the subject contract and relax the triceps muscle to ensure than no muscle is included in the fold. Hold the fold firmly and do not release it until the measurement has been read.

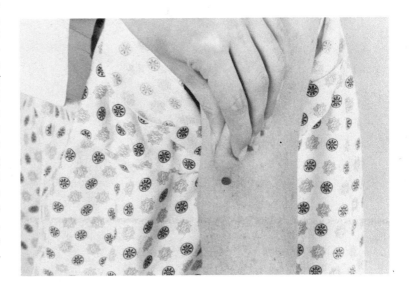

2. Pick up the calipers with the right hand and depress the spring loaded lever. Apply the caliper jaws over the fat fold exactly at the midpoint of the arm at a depth about equal to the thickness of the fold. Place the caliper jaws on the fold below the fingers so that pressure is exerted by the calipers and not the fingers.

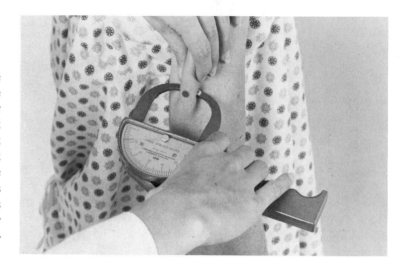

3. Release the spring loaded lever while holding the fold. Read measurement approximately two seconds after full pressure is applied to the skinfold. Depress the spring loaded lever and remove calipers.

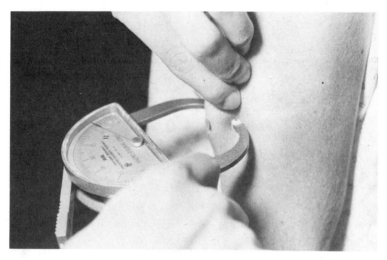

4. Repeat steps 1-4 two more times and record all measurements. Average the three skinfold measurements and record the average on the Nutritional Assessment Data Card or Record (Figs. 1 and 4).

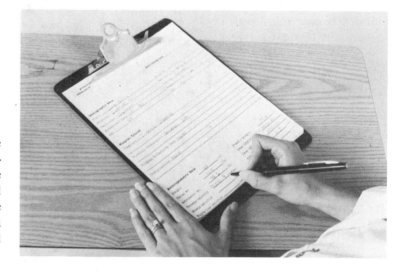

REPORTING AND RECORDING

1. Record all anthropometric measurements on the Screening Nutritional Assessment Data Card or the Profile Data Record.
2. Return completed Data Cards and Records to the Nutritional Assessment Center.

REFERENCES

1. Durnin, J.V. and Womersley, J.: Body fat assessed from total body density and its estimation from skinfold thickness: Measurements on 481 men and women aged from 16 to 72 years. Br. J. Nutr. 32:77, 1974.
2. Frisancho, A.R.: Triceps skinfold and upper arm muscle size: Norms for assessment of nutritional status. Am. J. Clin. Nutr. 27:1052, 1974.
3. Jelliffe, D.B.: Direct nutritional assessment of human groups, in The Assessment of Nutritional Status of the Community. Geneva, Switzerland: World Health Organization, 1966, pp. 238-239.
4. Lindner, P. and Lindner, D.: How to assess degrees of fatness: A working manual, 1973.
5. Ruiz, L., Colley, J.R. and Hamilton, P.J.: Measurement of triceps skinfold thickness: An investigation of sources of variation. Br. J. Prev. Soc. Med. 25:165, 1971.
6. Weiner, J.S. and Lourie, J.A.: Anthropometry, in Human Biology. A Guide to Field Methods, IBP Handbook No. 9, Oxford: Blackwell Scientific Publication, 1969, pp. 4-35.
7. Zerfas, A.J.: The insertion tape: A new circumference tape for use in nutritional assessment. Am. J. Clin. Nutr. 28:782, 1975.

G. Procedure for Measuring Arm Circumference and Triceps Skinfold in the Supine Position

PURPOSE

The purposes of the procedure for measuring triceps skinfold and arm circumference in the supine position are:

1. To define techniques for measuring triceps skinfold and arm circumference accurately, reproducibly and comparably when the patient is unable to assume the recommended upright stance for measurement.
2. To assess the status of body fat and somatic protein stores.
3. To identify those patients who are nutritionally at risk.
4. To evaluate patient response to nutrition therapy.

GENERAL INFORMATION

1. Due to injury, traction and/or disease, many patients may be unable to assume the recommended upright stance for anthropometric measurements. These patients might include those with major burns, multiple trauma and closed head injuries.
2. Since these patients may experience severe skeletal muscle depletion due to immobility, serial assessment of fat and skeletal muscle stores is particularly important.
3. All anthropometric measurements are performed by nutrition technicians from the Department of Dietetics, Nutritional Assessment Program. All initial and serial measurements on a given patient will be performed by the same technician when possible to ensure the most accurate and comparable measurements.
4. Procedural steps are very similar to those defined in Section II-F except that patient position is altered. Refer to this procedure for further information.

EQUIPMENT

- Lange skinfold caliper with constant pressure of 10 g/sq mm
- Insertion tape
- Pen or pencil
- Data card or record
- Adhesive labels

PROCEDURE

Location of upper arm midpoint:

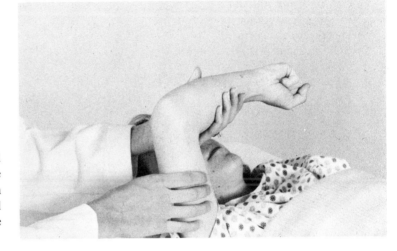

1. Instruct the patient to bend the right arm at a 90° angle from the elbow, lift the arm so that the elbow is pointed toward the ceiling and make a fist.

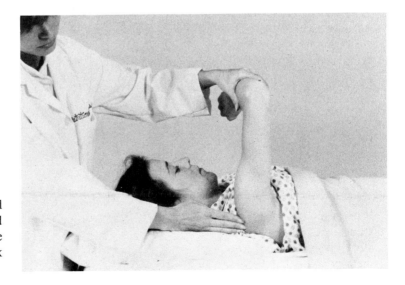

2. Locate the tip of the acromial process of the scapula and the olecranon process of the ulna by palpation and mark these sites while palpating.

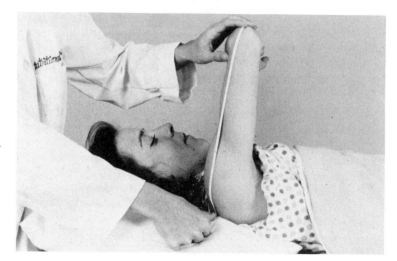

3. Place the zero inch mark of the insertion tape against the marked tip of the olecranon process and run the tape down the posterior side of the upper arm to the marked tip of the acromial process.

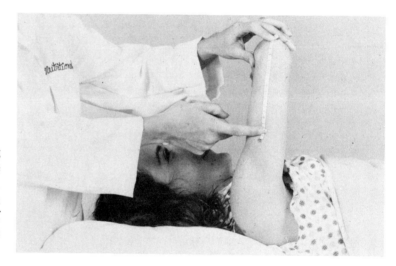

4. Loop the tape in half, joining the two measured ends at the tip of the olecranon process. Mark the midpoint with an adhesive label at the end of the loop directly in line with the olecranon process.

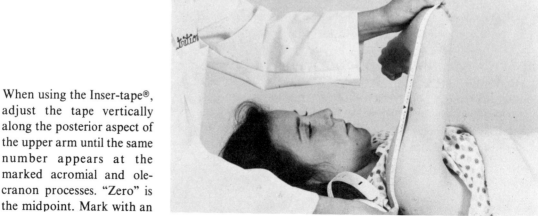

5. When using the Inser-tape®, adjust the tape vertically along the posterior aspect of the upper arm until the same number appears at the marked acromial and olecranon processes. "Zero" is the midpoint. Mark with an

6. Repeat steps 1-5 to ensure that the midpoint has been identified correctly.

Measurement of midupper arm circumference:

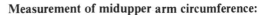

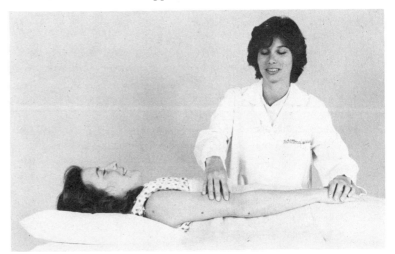

1. Instruct the patient to relax the right arm at his side while resting the right hand on the right thigh.

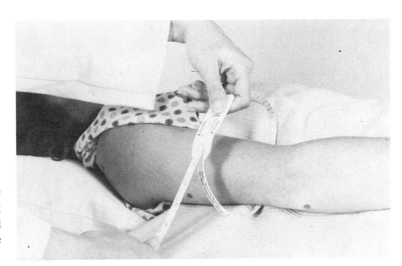

2. Slip the insertion tape around the patient's right arm and thread the distal end of the tape through the slot in the origin

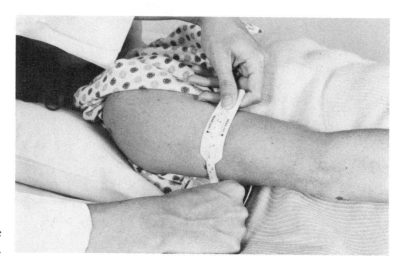

3. Align the upper edge of the tape with the midpoint mark.

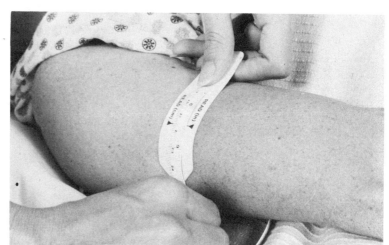

4. Tighten the tape until it is in contact with the skin without constricting it. Read the arm circumference through the window at the origin of the tape to the nearest 0.1 cm.

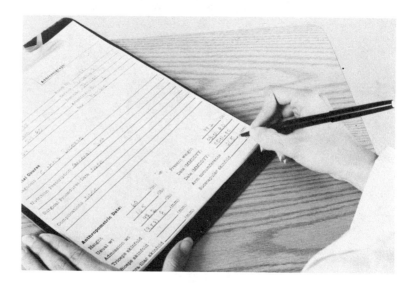

5. Record the measurement.

Measurement of triceps skinfold:

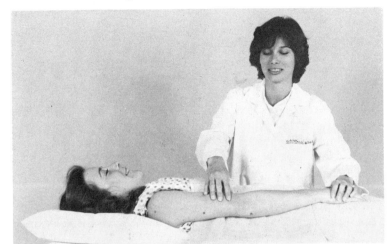

1. Measure the right arm while resting freely along the right side with the hand on the right thigh.

2. Pick up a lengthwise, vertical, double-fold of skin and fat about 1 cm above the midpoint mark, between the thumb and the forefinger of the left hand. The skinfold should be directly in line with the point of the olecranon process. Pull the skinfold cleanly away from underlying muscle. Have the subject contract and relax the triceps muscle to ensure that no muscle is included in the fold. Hold the fold firmly and do not release until the measurement has been read.

3. Pick up the calipers with the right hand and depress the spring loaded lever. Apply caliper jaws over the fat fold exactly at the midpoint of the arm to a depth about equal to the thickness of the fold. Place the caliper jaws on the fold below the fingers so that pressure is exerted by the calipers and not the fingers.

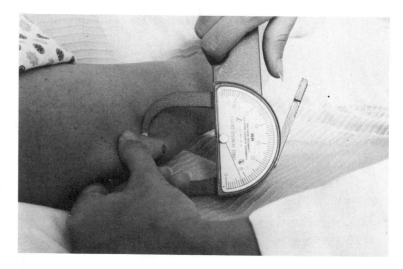

4. Release the spring loaded lever while holding the fold. Read the measurement approximately two seconds after full pressure is applied to the skinfold. Depress the spring loaded lever and remove calipers.

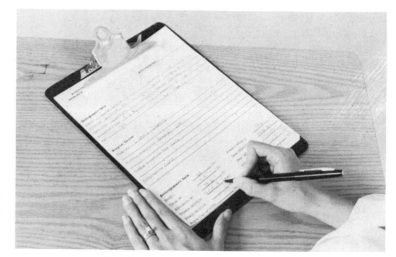

5. Record the measurement to the nearest mm on the Nutritional Assessment Data Card or Record (see Figs. 1 and 4).

Repeat steps 1-5 two more times and record measurements. Average the three recorded skinfold measurements and record the average on the Nutritional Assessment Data Card or Record.

REPORTING AND RECORDING

1. Record anthropometric measurements on the Screening Nutritional Assessment Data Card or Profile Data Record.

2. Return completed Data Cards or Records to the Nutritional Assessment Center.

REFERENCE

1. Jensen, T.G., Dudrick, S.J. and Johnston, D.: A comparison of triceps skinfold and arm circumference values measured in standard and supine positions. JPEN 3:513, 1979.

H. Procedure for Calibrating
Lange Skinfold Calipers _____

PURPOSE

The purposes of the procedure for calibrating the Lange skinfold calipers are:

1. To routinely check skinfold caliper pressure over the entire operating range of measurements.
2. To ensure accuracy of skinfold measurements.

GENERAL INFORMATION

1. Caliper pressure of 10 g/sq mm is preferable to very low or high pressures and all calipers must be calibrated at this pressure to ensure accuracy and reproducibility of skinfold measurements.
2. The Standards for Anthropometric Measurements from the Health and Nutritional Examination Survey, which are currently used for data analysis, were derived from skinfold measurements taken with Lange® calipers having a pressure of 10 g/mm² of contact surface area. All data compared with these standards must be obtained using identical methodology for purposes of standardization and accurate interpretation.
3. Caliper pressure must be constant over the range of jaw openings from 10 to at least 50 mm with a contact surface from 10 to 50 mm.
4. The Lange skinfold caliper is a reliable precision instrument when used properly. However, calibration will be destroyed by adverse environmental conditions and/or indiscriminant handling. The following situations commonly affect calibration of the caliper:
   a. Dropping the caliper.
   b. Storing in humid environment.
   c. Storing in dirty environment.
   d. Depressing the spring loaded lever unnecessarily.
5. Since humidity and dirt may adversely affect the caliper lubricant and calibration, each caliper must be stored and carried in the

individual case supplied with the unit at all times when not in use. In addition, the calipers must be stored overnight in the specified place and never taken outside the air-conditioned hospital environment.

6. The caliper must be used only according to defined procedure to prevent unnecessary manipulation (see Sections II-F and II-G).

7. Accuracy of the caliper must be tested on a monthly basis and is done using a specially designed calibration block. The calibration block is a metal device consisting of the following parts (Fig. 14):

   a. Step 1: The first step of the block tests calibration at the 10 mm jaw opening level. The caliper scale should read 10 mm when the jaws are applied to this step if the calipers are precisely calibrated.

   b. Step 2: The second step of the block tests calibration at the 20 mm jaw opening level. The caliper scale should read 20 mm when the jaws are applied to this step if the calipers are precisely calibrated.

   c. Step 3: The third step of the block tests calibration at the 30 mm jaw opening level. The caliper scale should read 30 mm when the jaws are applied to this step if the calipers are precisely calibrated.

   d. Step 4: The fourth step of the block tests calibration at the 40 mm jaw opening level. The caliper scale should read 40 mm when the jaws are applied to this step if the calipers are precisely calibrated.

   e. Step 5: The fifth step of the block tests calibration at the 50 mm jaw opening level. The caliper scale should read 50 mm when the jaws are applied to this step if the calipers are precisely calibrated.

8. Lange® calipers are tested on a weekly basis by the secretarial coordinator of the Nutritional Assessment Program.

9. For practical purposes, Lange calipers are considered to be in calibration if the scale reading is within 0.5 mm of the desired stepwise reading when caliper jaws are applied at full pressure.

10. Any caliper which is not properly calibrated must be returned immediately to Cambridge Scientific Industries, P.O. Box 265, Moose Lodge Road, Cambridge, Maryland 21613. Type of repair must be indicated on work order as calibrating, cleaning, lubricating, or replacing crystal.

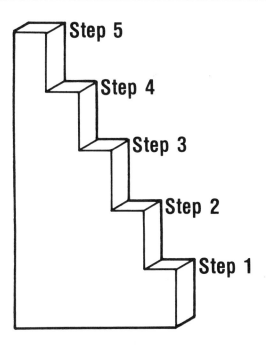

Figure 14. Calibration Block. Accuracy of the skinfold caliper is tested with a calibration block.

EQUIPMENT

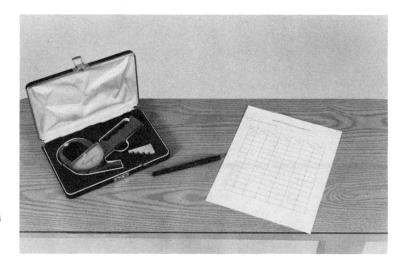

- Lange skinfold caliper
- Calibration block
- Skinfold Caliper Calibration Record
- Pen or pencil

PROCEDURE

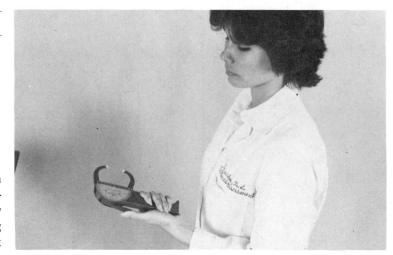

1. Grasp the caliper handle in the left hand so that the caliper face and scale are clearly visible. Depress the spring loaded lever with the left thumb.

2. Insert step 1 of the calibration block between the open jaws, while holding the block in the right hand between thumb and forefinger. Release spring loaded lever with thumb of left hand and read the caliper scale at eye level two seconds after full pressure is applied. Record caliper reading on the Skinfold Caliper Calibration Record (Fig. 15). If the needle points between 9.5 mm and 10.5 mm on face scale, caliper is properly calibrated at the 10 mm jaw opening level.

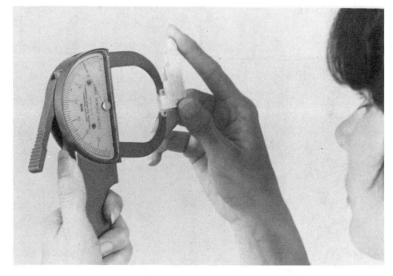

3. Depress the spring loaded lever with thumb of left hand and apply caliper jaws to step
 • 2 of the calibration block. Release the spring loaded lever with left thumb and read caliper scale at eye level two seconds after full pressure is applied. Record the reading on the Skinfold Caliper Calibration Record. If the needle points between 19.5 and 20.5 mm on the caliper scale, the caliper is properly calibrated at the 20 mm jaw opening level.

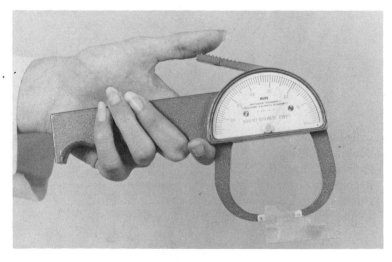

SKINFOLD CALIPER CALIBRATION RECORD

Caliper Identification Number: _____

Date	Step 1 mm	Step 2 mm	Step 3 mm	Step 4 mm	Step 5 mm	Initials

Figure 15. Skinfold Caliper Calibration Record. Calibration measurements are taken weekly and recorded on the Skinfold Caliper Calibration Record.

4. Depress the spring loaded lever with the thumb of the left hand and apply the caliper jaws to step 3 of the calibration block. Release the spring loaded lever with the thumb of the left hand and read the caliper scale at eye level two seconds after full pressure is applied. Record the measurement on the Skinfold Caliper Calibration Record. If the needle points between 29.5 and 30.5 on the caliper scale, the caliper is properly calibrated at the 30

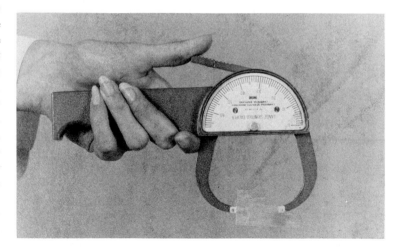

5. Depress the spring loaded lever again in the same manner. Apply the caliper jaws to the fourth step of the calibration block. Release the spring loaded lever with the thumb of the left hand and read the caliper scale at eye level two seconds after full pressure is applied. Record the reading on the Skinfold Caliper Calibration Record. If the needle points between 39.5 and 40.5 on the caliper scale, the caliper is properly calibrated at the 40 mm jaw opening level.

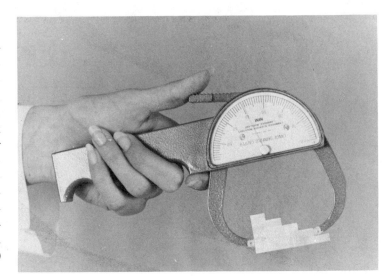

6. Depress spring loaded lever again in the same manner. Apply caliper jaws to the fifth step of the calibration block. Release spring loaded lever with thumb of left hand and read the caliper scale at eye level two seconds after full pressure is applied. Record the reading on the Skinfold Caliper Calibration Record. If the needle points between 49.5 and 50.5, caliper is properly calibrated.

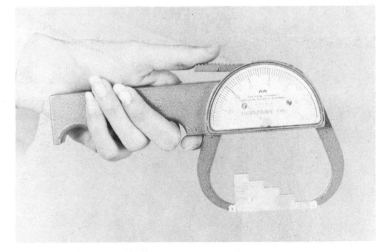

7. Return the Lange skinfold calipers and calibrating block to the individual carrying case. Initial and date the Skinfold Caliper Calibration Record and return it to the appropriate file.

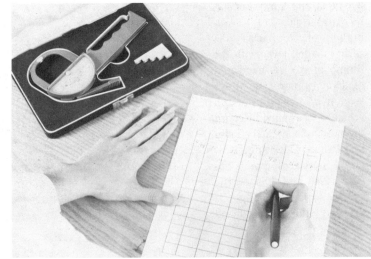

REPORTING AND RECORDING

1. Record the caliper identification number, date and all calibration measurements taken on the Skinfold Caliper Calibration Record.
2. Report any caliper which needs adjustment to the program coordinator immediately.

REFERENCE

1. Cambridge Scientific Industries (Ron Moore, National Sales Manager): Personal communication.

I. Procedure for Initiating Food and Fluid Intakes

PURPOSE

The purposes of the procedure for initiating food and fluid intakes are:

1. To ensure that materials for recording food and fluid intakes are properly disseminated and readily available.
2. To ensure that the patient and nursing staff understand the procedure for recording food and fluid intakes and cooperate during the recording period.

GENERAL INFORMATION

1. Energy and nutrient intakes are calculated from food and fluid intake records on a daily basis as a serial component of the Nutritional Assessment Program.
2. Food and fluid intake records are initiated by nutrition technicians from the Department of Dietetics, Nutritional Assessment Program.
3. Food and fluid intakes are initiated the day before the actual recording procedure is to begin.

EQUIPMENT

- Opaque adhesive tape
- Pen or pencil
- Black marker
- Ten Nutrient Intake Records/ Oral Food and Fluids and/or Ten Nutrient Intake Records/ Enteral Formulas, IVH Solutions, IV Fluids
- Calorie Intake and Weight Record
- Nutritional Assessment Menu Envelope

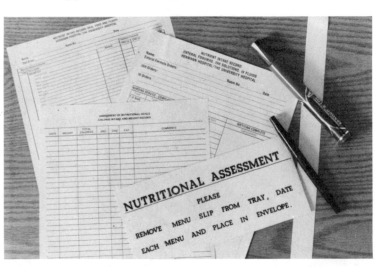

PROCEDURE

NUTRIENT INTAKE RECORD/ORAL FOOD AND FLUIDS
HERMANN HOSPITAL/THE UNIVERSITY HOSPITAL

Name: _Jane Doe_   Room No. _4427_   Date _3-3-81_
Diet Order: _General diet - six small feedings_

Nursing Service Complete			Dietitian Complete		
Time	Description	Amount	PRO (g)	CHO (g)	FAT (g)
	BREAKFAST				
	Juice of Fruit				
	Cereal				
	Egg				
	Meat				
	Beverage(s)				
	Milk				
	Margarine				
	Sugar				
	Breakfast Bread				
	Other				
	BETWEEN MEAL FEEDING				
	(Snacks and/or Supplements)				

1. Review all current nutrition orders for the patient in the Physician's Order section of the medical record. Select the appropriate Nutrient Intake Record. The Nutrient Intake Record/Oral Foods and Fluids and/or Nutrient Intake Record/ Enteral Formulas, IVH Solutions, IV Fluids may be selected (Figs. 16 and 17).

Complete the following information on ten of each of the Nutrient Intake Records:

    a. Patient name.
    b. Room number.
    c. Date.
    d. Nutrition orders.

2. Attach the Nutrient Intake Records and Calorie Intake and Weight Record (Fig. 9) to the door of the patient's room with opaque adhesive tape. Label the adhesive tape with the Black marker as follows: NOTE: Record All Food and Fluid Intake. NOTE: Record Daily Weight.

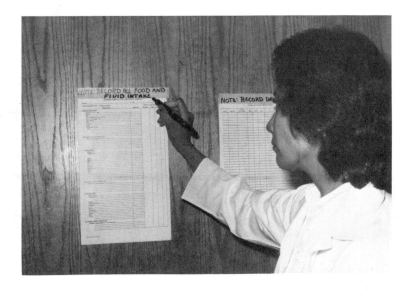

NUTRIENT INTAKE RECORD/ORAL FOOD AND FLUIDS
HERMANN HOSPITAL/THE UNIVERSITY HOSPITAL

Name: _____ Room No. _____ Date _____

Diet Order: _____

Nursing Service Complete			Dietitian Complete			
Time	Description	Amount	PRO (g)	CHO (g)	FAT (g)	Other
	BREAKFAST					
	Juice of Fruit _____					
	Cereal _____					
	Egg _____					
	Meat _____					
	Beverage(s) _____					
	Milk _____					
	Margarine _____					
	Sugar _____					
	Breakfeast Bread _____					
	Other _____					
	_____					
	_____					
	_____					
	_____					
	BETWEEN MEAL FEEDING					
	(Snacks and/or Supplements) _____					
	_____					
	_____					
	_____					
	LUNCH					
	Entree _____					
	Vegetable(s) _____					
	Vegetable(s)					
	Vegetable(s)					
	Salad _____					
	Salad Dressing _____					
	Dessert _____					
	Fruit _____					
	Bread _____					
	Margarine _____					
	Sugar _____					
	Beverage _____					
	Milk _____					
	Other _____					
	_____					
	_____					
	BETWEEN MEAL FEEDING					
	(Snacks and/or Supplements) _____					
	_____					
	_____					
	_____					
	DINNER					
	Entree _____					
	Vegetable(s) _____					
	Vegetable(s)					
	Vegetable(s)					
	Salad _____					
	Salad Dressing _____					
	Dessert _____					
	Fruit _____					
	Bread _____					
	Margarine _____					
	Sugar _____					
	Beverage _____					
	Milk _____					
	Other _____					
	_____					
	_____					
	BETWEEN MEAL FEEDING					
	(Snacks and/or Supplements) _____					
	_____					
	_____					
	_____					
	TOTAL					
			× 4	× 4	× 9	

TOTAL CALORIES = _____ + _____ + _____ = _____

Figure 16. Nutrient Intake Record/Oral Food and Fluids. All orally consumed foods and fluids are recorded by staff nurses on designated record forms which are subsequently collected by nutrition technicians for energy nutrient calculations.

NUTRIENT INTAKE RECORD
ENTERAL FORMULAS, IVH SOLUTIONS, IV FLUIDS
HERMANN HOSPITAL/THE UNIVERSITY HOSPITAL

Name: _____ Room No. _____ Date _____

Enteral Formula Orders: _____

IVH Orders: _____

IV Orders: _____

NURSING SERVICE - COMPLETE			DIETITIAN COMPLETE
Time	Type of Formula or Solution	Volume (cc)	Calculations
7-3 Shift 7:00 a.m.			
8:00 a.m.			
9:00 a.m.			
10:00 a.m.			
11:00 a.m.			
12:00 p.m.			
1:00 p.m.			
2:00 p.m.			
3-11 Shift 3:00 p.m.			
4:00 p.m.			
5:00 p.m.			
6:00 p.m.			
7:00 p.m.			
8:00 p.m.			
9:00 p.m.			
10:00 p.m.			
11-7 Shift 11:00 p.m.			
12:00 a.m.			
1:00 a.m			
2:00 a.m.			
3:00 a.m.			
4:00 a.m.			
5:00 a.m.			
6:00 a.m.			
TOTAL			

Figure 17. Nutrient Intake Record/Enteral formulas, IVH solutions, IV fluids. All enteral and parenteral fluids administered are recorded by staff nurses on this record form which is subsequently collected by nutrition technicians for nutrient calculations.

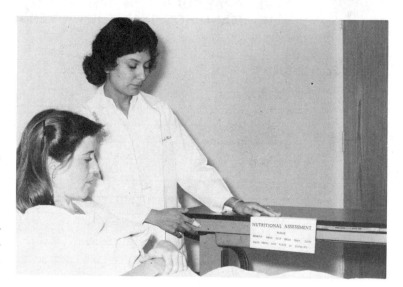

3. Attach the Nutritional Assessment Menu Envelope to the patients bedside table with adhesive tape (Fig. 18). Instruct the patient to save all menus from meal service trays and place them in the envelope.

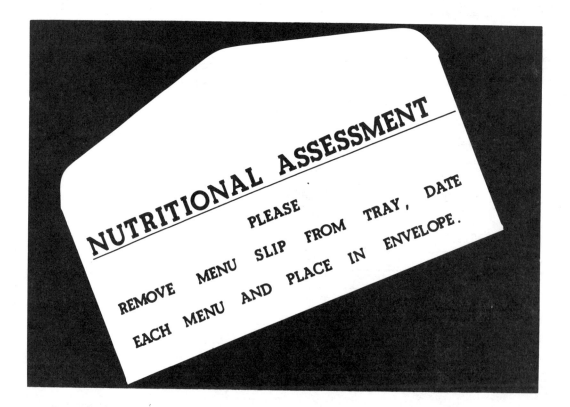

Figure 18. Nutritional Assessment Menu Envelope. The menu envelope is placed at the patient's bedside to facilitate collection of menus from meal trays for checking the accuracy of intake records.

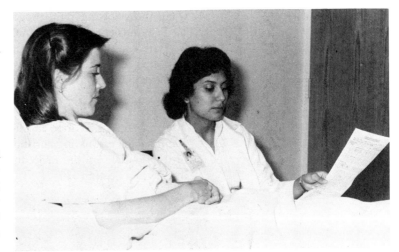

4. Explain the purpose of the Nutrient Intake Records and the procedure for recording food and fluid intakes correctly to the patient and the primary nurse (see Section II-J).

Jane Doe		21	2/29/81
PATIENT NAME		AGE	ADM. DATE

General diet - six small feeding
Ensure Plus - 150 ml TID

Record food and fluid intake

FLUIDS:

FORCE
RESTRICT
7 - 3
3 - 11
11 - 7

O · RT.   Q
IETER   IV   WT.

URINE TESTING

E   LAB   DATE   X - RAY PROCEDURES

5. Check the nursing cardex to ensure that "record food and fluid intake" is written as part of the diet order.

PATIENT'S
HISTORY, PHYSICAL AND PROGRESS NOTES
HERMANN HOSPITAL/*The University Hospital*

DATE OF SERVICE

DATE & TIME	
6-1-81	Nutritional Assessment Note:
	Nutrient intake has been initiated. Calculated
	protein, carbohydrate, fat and energy intakes will be
	recorded daily beginning 6-3-81 for the previous
	24-hour period
	Terri Jensen, M.S., R.D (J.D)

6. Chart that nutrient intake has been initiated in the progress notes of the Medical Record.

RECORDING AND REPORTING

1. Chart the following in the progress notes of the medical record:
   a. That nutrient intake was initiated.
   b. Date nutrient intakes will begin and be recorded in the chart.
   c. Name of the dietitian followed by the initials of technician in parentheses.

PATIENT TEACHING

1. Inform patient that food and fluid intake records are useful for planning and evaluating nutrition care.
2. Instruct patient on the Procedure for Recording Food and Fluid Intakes (see Section II-J).

J. Procedure for Recording Food and Fluid Intakes

The purposes of the procedure for recording food and fluid intakes are:

1. To provide an accurate record of foods and fluids ingested and/or administered over a 24-hour time period.
2. To maintain accurate records for calculation of daily energy and nutrient intakes and nitrogen balance.
3. To provide an objective basis for evaluating nutritional therapy.

1. Food and fluid intakes are recorded daily from 7:00 A.M. to 7:00 A.M. the following day by nursing personnel for all patients on nutritional assessment.
2. Daily intakes of calories, protein, carbohydrate and fat are calculated from these records. In addition, nitrogen intake is compared with nitrogen excretion to determine nitrogen balance every ten days. This objective data provides guidelines for altering nutrition therapy and interpreting changes in body weight.
3. Nitrogen balance compares nitrogen ingested with nitrogen excreted in the urine for an estimation of nitrogen retention. If intake is being recorded for nitrogen balance determination, a simultaneous 24-hour urine specimen must also be collected (see Section II-M).
4. Intravenous fluids, intravenous hyperalimentation solutions and enteral formulas contain these nutrients and must be recorded when administered during the recording period.
5. If any food or fluid which contains nutrients is consumed or administered and not simultaneously recorded, the record will not reflect actual 24-hour intake, and all calculations and test results will be invalid.
6. A complete record, therefore, requires total understanding and

cooperation from the patient and all nursing personnel involved in the patient's care during the recording period.

7. Recording consumed foods and fluids and all administered enteral and parenteral fluids is the responsibility of the staff nurse assigned to the patient. Supervision and coordination of the 24-hour intake record during nursing shift changes is the responsibility of the charge nurse.

8. Forms for recording nutrient intakes will be distributed to patient rooms prior to the initiation of the procedure and collected at the end of the 24-hour recording period by nutrition technicians from the Department of Dietetics, Nutritional Assessment Program.

9. Oral, enteral and parenteral nutrient intakes will be calculated and recorded in the progress notes of the medical record within 12 hours after the conclusion of the recording period.

10. Fluid intakes are recorded in cubic centimeters (cc). Foods which are liquid at room temperature are also considered fluid. Fluid capacities of measurement units and containers used in the hospital are as follows:

Container of juice	120 cc
Container of ice tea	240 cc
Container of milk	240 cc
Container of coffee	140 cc
Bottle of coke	180 cc
Dish of jello	120 cc
Carton of ice cream or sherbet	45 cc
Bowl of cooked cereal	110 cc
Bowl of soup	90 cc
1/4 teaspoon	1 cc
1 teaspoon	4 cc
1 ounce	30 cc
1 cup	240 cc
1 pint	480 cc
1 quart	960 cc

11. *Accuracy* is the key element in this procedure.

EQUIPMENT

- Nutrient Intake Record/Oral Foods and Fluids
- Nutrient Intake Record/Enteral Formulas, IVH Solutions, IV Fluids
- Pen or pencil
- Graduated container calibrated in cubic centimeters
- Nutritional Assessment Envelope

PROCEDURE

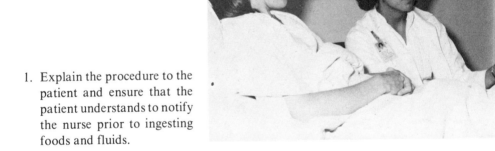

1. Explain the procedure to the patient and ensure that the patient understands to notify the nurse prior to ingesting foods and fluids.

2. Record all orally consumed food on the appropriate record for the 24-hour period beginning at 7:00 A.M. and ending at 7:00 A.M. the following day as follows:

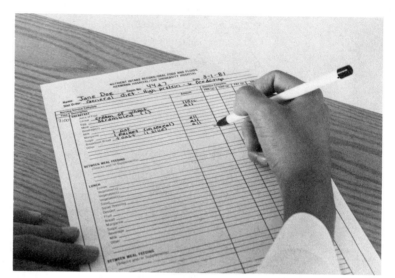

   a. Identify the food or fluid item correctly and describe as precisely as possible, i.e., *roast* beef, *2 percent lowfat* milk, *orange* sherbet, *fried* chicken.

   b. Record amounts of all foods consumed in fractions of portion measures, i.e., all, 3/4, 2/3, 1/2, 1/3, 1/4, 1/8.

   c. Note the approximate time of food or fluid intake.

3. Measure and record all orally consumed fluids on the appropriate record as follows:

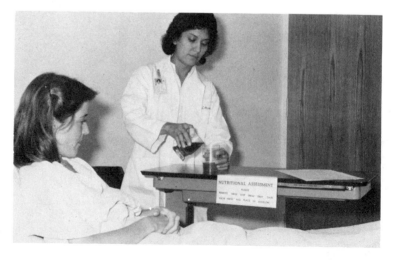

   a. Transfer all beverages to the graduated container and note the initial volume.

   b. After ingestion of fluid subtract the remaining volume from the initial volume and record the difference in cc.

   c. Note the time of fluid ingestion.

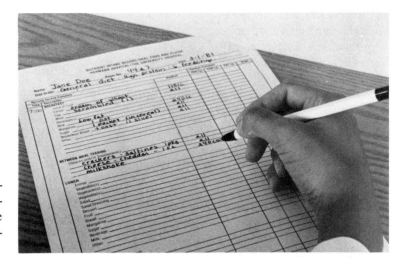

4. Record food and/or fluid ingested between meals or during the night in the same manner in the space provided.

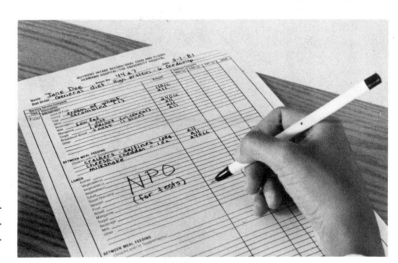

5. If the patient is NPO or refuses food record this information on the Nutrient Intake Record.

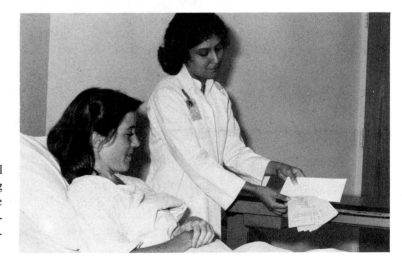

6. Save all menus from meal trays during the recording period and place them in the Nutritional Assessment Envelope attached to the bedside table.

7. If the patient is receiving IV fluids, intravenous hyperalimentation solutions or enteral formulas record the volume actually administered in ml per hour on the appropriate form as follows:

a. Identify the type of fluid, i.e., ensure tube feeding, IV D_5W, or IVH-1L 500 ml $D_{50}W$ + 500 ml FreAmine.

b. Record volume actually administered during the hour in ml.

c. Also record all fat emulsions, albumin or other intermittently administered fluid.

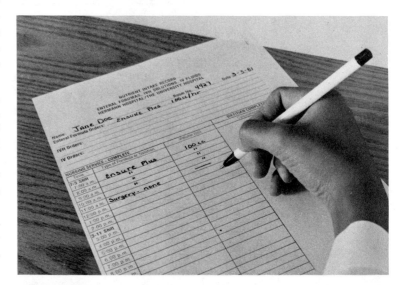

8. Total the 24-hour volume of fluid administered at the end of the recording period.

RECORDING AND REPORTING

1. Record all oral food and fluid intake on the Nutrient Intake Record/Oral Food and Fluids.

2. Record all administered fluids on the Nutrient Intake Record/Enteral Formulas, Intravenous Hyperalimentation Solutions and IV fluids.

3. Chart any problem or error which might cause intake records to be incomplete or inaccurate. Also record on Nutrient Intake Records.

4. Chart any suggestions for increasing oral intake.

PATIENT TEACHING

1. Explain the entire procedure and purposes of the procedure to the patient and ensure understanding. Patient cooperation is essential.
2. Instruct patient to save all menus and place them in the Nutritional Assessment Envelope.
3. Instruct the patient to notify the nurse prior to ingestion of foods and fluids.
4. Explain the purpose and use of the graduate container and instruct patient to drink all fluids directly from the graduate.

REFERENCE

1. Leaky M.J.: Measuring and recording fluid intake and output, in A Manual of Simple Nursing Procedures. Philadelphia: W.B. Saunders, 1971, pp. 64-68.

K. Procedure for Calculating Energy and Nutrient Intakes _____

PURPOSE

The purposes of the procedure for calculating energy and nutrient intakes are:

1. To determine the approximate energy and nutrient composition of food and fluid ingested and/or administered in the 24-hour recording period.
2. To determine nitrogen intake for computation of nitrogen balance.
3. To provide an objective basis for changing and coordinating enteral and/or parenteral nutritional therapy.

GENERAL GUIDELINES

1. Nutrient Intake Records are collected daily from patient rooms by nutrition technicians from the Department of Dietetics, Nutritional Assessment Program.
2. Nutrient intakes are calculated on a daily basis for the preceding 24-hour period from 7:00 A.M. to 7:00 A.M.
3. Daily intakes of carbohydrate, protein, fat and calories are routinely calculated. However, other nutrients may also be included at the request of the physician and/or clinical dietitian.
4. Energy and nutrient calculations may be ascertained in two ways:
   a. By entering recorded data into the computer terminal which is programmed to generate a complete nutritional analysis.
   b. By using handbooks of food composition to determine nutrient content for individual items and then calculating total intake on a pocket calculator.
   Although the latter method is the most time consuming and laborious, this procedure will define the method for hand calculation since this skill is essential when the computer is temporarily unavailable or an unusual intake is required.
5. Calculated nutrient/energy intakes are estimates since actual con-

sumption is approximated and because food samples may vary in composition. However, estimated energy/nutrient intakes are of great value in evaluating changes in nutritional status when considered with other clinical and biochemical data.

6. Energy and nutrient content data for foods and beverages served in this hospital are based on manufacturer's analysis when possible.

7. Recipe calculations are based on nutritive data from *Food Values of Portions Commonly Used* by Church and Church which are adapted to portion sizes used in this hospital.

8. Nutrient composition data for commercial enteral formulas and IV solutions is much more precise, since exact nutrient composition is known. All cited data are based on manufacturer's analysis.

9. The following factors are used to calculate calories per gram of nutrient:

Dextrose	3.4 calories/g
Carbohydrate	4 calories/g
Protein	4 calories/g
Fat	9 calories/g

10. Nitrogen intake is determined by dividing the protein intake by 6.25, since nitrogen accounts for 16 percent of the protein molecule.

11. Average protein and calorie intakes are calculated every ten days for the previous ten-day period, since frequent diagnostic and surgical procedures may complicate accurate assessment and interpretation of daily calculations.

12. The key element in this procedure is *accuracy* both in recording and calculating data.

EQUIPMENT

- Completed Nutrient Intake Record(s)
- Pen or pencil
- Pocket calculator
- Calorie Intake and Weight Record
- Food Composition References

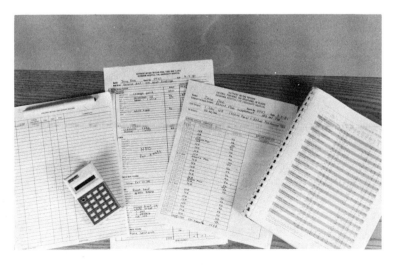

PROCEDURE

1. Obtain the previous day's Nutrient Intake Record(s) and menus from the patient's room and review the recorded intake and menus with the patient to ensure that *all* intake has been accurately recorded for the previous 24-hour period. Then review the nurse's notes and intake and output records for the previous day and compare with Nutrient Intake Records. Note any discrepancies and resolve with the nurse.

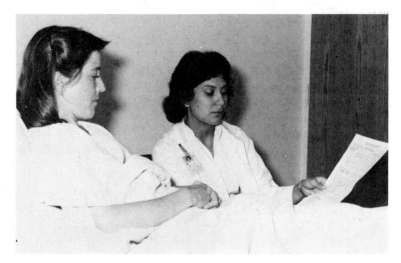

2. Calculate nutrient and energy intake of orally consumed foods and beverages by first determining protein (g), carbohydrate (g) and fat (g) content using appropriate references:

   a. Use the *Hermann Hospital Diet Reference Manual* as a reference for menu items. Refer to *Food Values of Portions Commonly Used* (Church and Church) for items brought in by friends and family. Consult with the clinical dietitian to determine the nutrient composition of unusual food items since a variety of other references are also available.[1-10]

   b. Record the carbohydrate, protein and fat content of each item in grams in the appropriate space on the Nutrient Intake Record. If fractions of portions are recorded, divide each cited number by the denominator of the fraction and multiply by the numerator to adjust calculations appropriately.

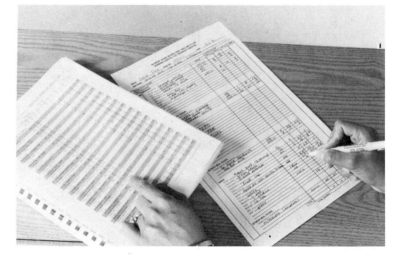

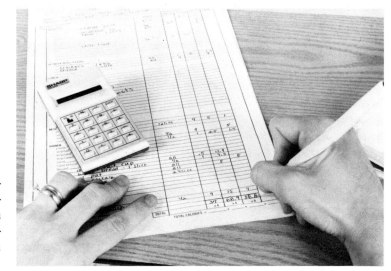

3. Determine the total nutrient intake of carbohydrate, protein and fat from oral foods and fluids by adding all numbers in each column.

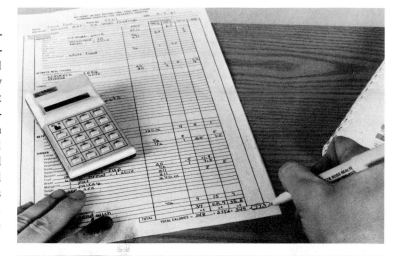

4. To determine the daily caloric intake, multiply the total grams of protein and carbohydrate consumed by four and total grams of fat consumed by nine (calories/g). Add calories from carbohydrate, protein and fat sources to calculate total caloric intake from oral foods and fluids. If this number is a fraction, round it off to the nearest whole number.

5. To calculate nutrient intake from commercial enteral products and formulas, first determine protein (g), fat (g) and carbohydrate (g) content per 100 ml of formula or 1 tablespoon of powder (Tables 1, 2, and 3).

TABLE 1. NUTRITIONAL SUPPLEMENTS

Product/Manufacturer	Protein (g)	Carbohydrate (g)	Fat (g)	Calories
Amin-Aid/McGaw	1.94	32.4	7.03	200
Citrotein/Doyle	4.0	12.2	0.2	66.3
Eggnog/Delmark	6.25	15.42	3.75	120.8
Hepatic-Aid/McGaw	4.26	28.7	3.6	165
Instant Breakfast Carnation	5.66	13.2	3.0	106
Lonalac/Mead Johnson	3.54	5.0	3.64	67
Portagen/Mead Johnson	3.6	11.9	4.9	100
Sustacal Powder/Mead Johnson	8.1	18.2	3.3	133

Nutritional Analysis per 100 ml at standard dilution.

TABLE 2. MODULAR SUPPLEMENTS

Product/Manufacturer	Protein (g)	Carbohydrate (g)	Fat (g)	Calories
Cal Power/General Mills	0	62.5	0	228
Casec/Mead Johnson (tbsp)	4.1	0	Trace	17
Controlyte/Doyle (tbsp)	Trace	6.5	2.2	45
dp HIGH P.E.R. Protein/General Mills (tbsp)	5.0	0.5	0.2	24
EMF/Control Drugs (tbsp)	7.5	1.5	0	36
Gevral/Lederle (tbsp)	2.93	1.18	0.1	18.3
HyCal/Beecham	Trace	60.2	Trace	295
Lipomul-Oral/Upjohn	33.3	0.66	66.6	594
Lytren/Mead Johnson	0	7.8	0	31.2
MCT Oil/Mead Johnson	0	0	93.3	774
Microlipid/Organon	0	0	50.0	450
Moducal/Mead Johnson	0	50	0	200
Polycose Liquid/Ross	0	50	0	200
Polycose Powder/Ross (tbsp)	0	7.5	0	32
Pro-Mix/Nubro (tbsp)	10.0	0.5	0	42
Sumacal/Organon	0	50	0	200

Nutritional Analysis per 100 ml or tbsp.

TABLE 3. NUTRITIONALLY COMPLETE FORMULAS FOR ORAL OR TUBE FEEDING

Product/Manufacturer	Protein (g)	Carbohydrate (g)	Fat (g)	Calories
Compleat-B/Doyle	4.0	12.0	4.0	100
Compleat Modified/Doyle	4.3	14.0	3.7	106
Ensure/Ross	3.7	14.5	3.7	106
Ensure Plus/Ross	5.5	20.0	5.3	150
Flexical/Mead Johnson	2.2	15.4	3.4	100
Formula II/Cutter Medical	3.8	12.3	4.0	100
Isocal/Mead Johnson	3.4	13.0	4.4	106
Magnacal/Organon	7.0	25.0	8.0	200
Meritine Liquid/Doyle	6.0	11.5	3.3	100

(continued)

TABLE 3. (*Continued*)

Product/Manufacturer	Protein (g)	Carbohydrate (g)	Fat (g)	Calories
Meritine Powder/Doyle	6.9	11.9	3.5	107
Nutri-1000/Cutter Medical	3.8	10.6	5.2	110
Nutri-1000 LF/Cutter Medical	3.9	10.5	4.7	106
Osmolite/Ross	3.7	14.3	3.8	106
Precision HN/Doyle	4.4	21.6	0.13	105
Precision Isotonic/Doyle	2.9	14.4	3.0	96
Precision LR/Doyle	2.63	24.9	0.16	111
Renu/Organon	3.3	13.0	4.0	100
Sustacal LF/Mead Johnson	6.0	13.8	2.3	100
Sustagen/Mead Johnson	11.1	31.7	1.6	186
Travasorb HN/Travanol	3.0	19.0	1.33	100
Travasorb Liquid/Travanol	3.69	14.4	3.7	105
Travasorb MCT/Travanol	3.0	19.0	1.33	100
Travasorb Std/Travanol	3.0	19.0	1.33	100
Viapep/Cutter	2.5	17.6	2.5	100
Vital/Ross	4.2	18.5	1.0	100
Vitaneed/Organon	3.5	13.0	4.0	100
Vivonex HN/Eaton	4.3	21.1	0.1	100
Vivonex STD/Eaton	2.1	23.0	0.1	100

Nutritional Analysis per 100 ml (at standard dilution).

6. Divide the total volume of product consumed by 100 to determine the multiplication factor which is necessary to convert nutrient content per volume cited to that actually consumed. (For powdered products simply determine the number of tablespoons consumed.) Multiply the cited protein, fat and carbohydrate in grams by this factor to ascertain total intake of each nutrient.

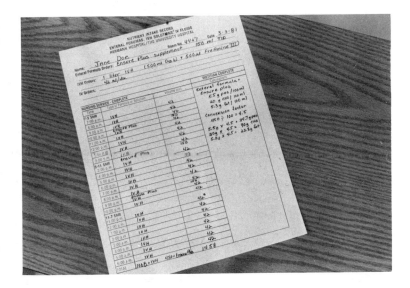

7. To determine the daily caloric intake from enteral formulas, multiply the total grams of protein and carbohydrate consumed by four and total grams of fat consumed by nine (calories/g). Add calories from carbohydrate, protein and fat sources.

8. To calculate intravenous nutrient intake, determine total milliliters actually infused over the 7:00 A.M. to 7:00 A.M. period for each of the following:
   a. IV dextrose (peripheral)
   b. IVH Base Solution (dextrose and amino acid solutions)
   c. Fat emulsion

9. Multiply the total infused volume for each component by the conversion factors (g nutrient per ml) listed in Table 4 to ascertain nutrient content of infusate(s) in grams.

TABLE 4.

Nutrient Intake Component		g Nutrient/ml		Cal/ml	
Aminosyn	3.5%	0.035	g protein	0.14	kcal
Aminosyn	5.%	.05	g protein	0.20	kcal
Aminosyn	7.%	0.07	g protein	0.308	kcal
Aminosyn	8.5%	0.085	g protein	0.34	kcal
Aminosyn	10%	0.01	g protein	0.398	kcal
FreAmine II	8.5%	0.078	g protein	0.312	kcal
FreAmine III	8.5%	.085	g protein	0.328	kcal
Travasol	5.5%	0.055	g protein	0.22	kcal
Travasol	8.5%	0.085	g protein	0.34	kcal
Veinamine	8.5%	0.072	g protein	0.288	kcal
Nephramine		0.051	g protein	0.146	kcal
Albumin		0.25	g protein	1.0	kcal
D_5W		0.05	g dextrose	0.262	kcal
$D_{10}W$		0.1	g dextrose	0.340	kcal
$D_{20}W$		0.2	g dextrose	0.680	kcal
$D_{30}W$		0.3	g dextrose	1.02	kcal
$D_{40}W$		0.4	g dextrose	1.36	kcal
$D_{50}W$		0.5	g dextrose	1.7	kcal
$D_{60}W$		0.6	g dextrose	2.04	kcal
$D_{70}W$		0.7	g dextrose	2.38	kcal
Intralipid	10%	0.12	g fat	1.1	kcal
Liposyn	10%	0.12	g fat	1.1	kcal

10. Multiply grams of infused dextrose by 3.4, protein by 4 and fat by 9 and add these subtotals to determine caloric intake from parenteral solutions and fluids.

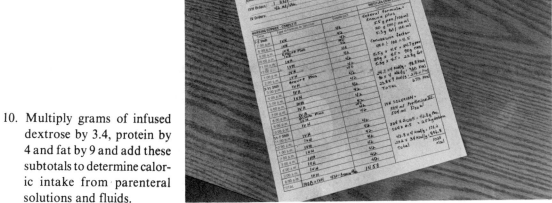

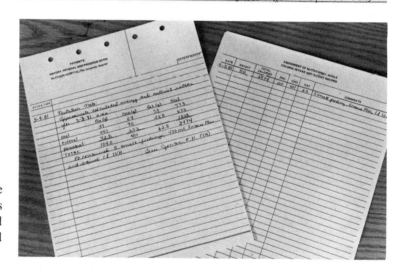

PATIENT'S
HISTORY, PHYSICAL AND PROGRESS NOTES
HERMANN HOSPITAL/*The University Hospital*

DATE OF SERVICE

DATE & TIME

3-4-81 | Nutrition Note:
Approximate calculated energy and nutrient intake
for 3-3-81 was:

	Pro (g)	CHO (g)	fat (g)	Kcal
oral	37	69	39	773
enteral	24.7	90	23.8	673
parenteral	42.8	252	—	1028
TOTAL	104.5	411	62.8	2474

Pt consumed 5 small feedings, 450 ml Ensure Plus
and received 1 l IVH.

Jean Jensen, R.D. (CH)

11. Add carbohydrate (g), protein (g), fat (g) and calories from all nutrient sources to determine the total daily intake.

12. Record calculations in the history and progress notes of the medical record and on the Nutrient Intake and Weight Record.

REPORTING AND RECORDING

1. Record total daily nutrient intake of carbohydrate (g), protein (g), fat (g) and calories on the Daily Nutrient Intake and Weight Record. Record sources of the intake under comments on this record, i.e., General diet—3 meals, 1000 ml Ensure Plus.

2. Record approximate nutrient intake of carbohydrate (g), protein (g), fat (g) and calories in the History and Progress notes of the Medical Record. Divide into oral, enteral, parenteral and total intake when possible.

   Information recorded in the Medical Record should include:

   a. Times and dates of recorded intake.

   b. Statement of exact content of nutritional intake, for example, General diet—three meals, 360 ml sustacal milkshake, 1 liter IVH with 25 g added albumin.

3. Sign the name of Clinical Dietitian Specialist with the nutrition technician's initials in parentheses following the name.

REFERENCES

1. Adams, C.: Nutritive value of American foods, Agriculture Handbook No. 456, U.S.D.A., Government Printing Office, 1976.
2. Appledorf, H.: Nutritional analysis of foods from fast-food-chains. Food Technol. 28:50, 1974.
3. Bridges, M. and Mattice, M.: Bridges Food and Beverage Analysis, 3rd edition, revised, Philadelphia: Lea and Ferbiger, 1950.
4. Church, C.F. and Church, H.N.: Food Values of Portions Commonly Used, 12th edition, revised, Philadelphia: J.B. Lippincott, 1975.
5. Feeley, R.M., Criner, P.E. and Watt, B.K.: Cholesterol content of foods. J. Am. Dietet. Assoc. 61:134, 1972.
6. Kilgore, L.: Proximate composition and energy value of pizza. J. Am. Dietet. Assoc. 50:133, 1967.
7. Posati, L. and Orr, M.: Composition of Foods, Agriculture Handbook No. 8-1 Dairy and Egg Products. U.S.D.A., Government Printing Office, 1976.
8. Watt, B.K. and Merrill, A.L.: Composition of Foods, Agriculture Handbook No. 8 U.S.D.A., Government Printing Office, 1963.
9. Watt, B.K., Gebhardt, S.E., et al.: Food composition tables for the 70s. J. Am. Dietet. Assoc. 6:257, 1974.
10. Nutritive Value of Foods, Home and Garden Bulletin, No. 72, Consumer and Food Economics Research Division, U.S.D.A. Government Printing Office, 1970.

L. Procedure for Ordering Laboratory Testing

PURPOSE

The purpose of the procedure for ordering laboratory testing is:

1. To ensure that all laboratory tests for nutritional assessment purposes are ordered correctly and on schedule.

GENERAL INFORMATION

1. The following laboratory tests may be ordered for nutritional assessment purposes and are specified on the Nutritional Assessment General Order Set:

   (S) pr.

   a. Serum albumin concentration.
   b. Serum transferrin concentration.
   c. Thyroxin-binding prealbumin.
   d. Retinol-binding protein.

   Hydrat'n

   e. Serum osmolarity.
   f. White blood cell count with differential for lymphocytes.
   g. 24-hour urine creatinine.
   h. 24-hour urine urea nitrogen.

   These tests are repeated at ten-day serial intervals until all results are within normal limits.

2. Serum albumin, transferrin, prealbumin, and retinol-binding protein concentrations indicate the status of the visceral protein compartment. These proteins have different half-lives and levels of sensitivity to nutritional deprivation. Determination of serum concentrations permits classification of degree of visceral protein depletion and the adequacy of nutritional intervention can be measured by serial determinations.

3. Serum transferrin, prealbumin and retinol-binding protein are measured by radial immunodiffusion in the Immunology Laboratory of The Department of Pathology.

4. Serum albumin concentration is measured in the Chemistry Lab-

oratory of the same department by a direct colorimetric procedure. An Automatic Clinical Analyzer (ACA) is used to measure albumin quantitatively in serum. This method is an adaption of the bromcresol green (BCG) dye-binding method and is well recognized as superior to other dye-binding techniques because of its specificity and freedom from drug interference.

5. Serum osmolarity is a reliable indicator of hydration status. Since dehydration causes elevated serum protein concentrations and rehydration may depress serum protein concentrations, this test is helpful for valid interpretation of data. Serum osmolarity is measured in the Chemistry Laboratory of the Department of Pathology using an advanced cryomatic osmometer.

6. A total lymphocyte count is calculated from the white blood cell count and differential for lymphocytes. A depressed total lymphocyte count is consistent with impaired cellular defense mechanisms and malnutrition.

7. The white blood cell count is determined by electronic counting in the Hematology Laboratory of the Department of Pathology. The differential for lymphocytes is determined manually or electronically by counting the number of lymphocytes in a 100-cell stained smear. When the white blood cell count with differential for lymphocytes is ordered, the complete hematology profile is frequently done since the difference in cost is marginal. The complete hematology profile also includes hemoglobin and hematocrit determination, and these results should be noted when available. They are frequently useful since iron deficiency anemia may cause elevated serum transferrin concentration.

8. Urinary levels of creatinine are dependent principally upon the extent of skeletal muscle catabolism, especially during protein depletion. The status of skeletal muscle (somatic) protein can, therefore, be estimated by determining a creatinine/height index. The creatinine/height index is defined as the 24-hour creatinine excretion of a patient divided by the expected 24-hour creatinine excretion of a normal adult of the same height.

9. Since nitrogen is the primary component that differentiates protein from other basic nutrient moieties, nitrogen balance is employed as an index of protein nutritional status. Because urea accounts for 80 to 90 percent of total nitrogen loss, nitrogen balance can be computed for clinical purposes as nitrogen intake minus (urine urea nitrogen +4). The latter factor accounts for stool and skin losses as well as nonurea urinary nitrogen loss.

10. An automatic clinical analyzer is used to quantitatively measure urinary creatinine and urea nitrogen from the 24-hour urine sample in the Chemistry Laboratory of the Department of Pathology.

11. The ranges of expected values for these tests have been established in the hospital laboratory for adult patients as follows:

Serum albumin	3.5 -	5.5 g/dl
Serum transferrin	200 -	355 mg/dl

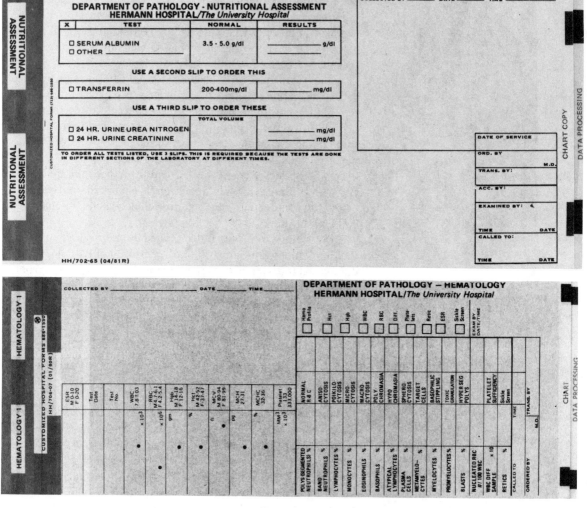

Figure 19. Nutritional Assessment Laboratory Requisitions. The use of specially designed laboratory requisitions permits results of laboratory tests to be delivered directly to the Nutritional Assessment Center.

Prealbumin	20 -	50 mg/dl
Retinol-binding protein	30 -	44 mcg/ml
Serum osmolarity	275 -	295 mOsm/l
White blood cell count	5800 -	10,800 cells/mm^3
Differential for lymphocytes	15%	
Urinary creatinine	20-26 mg/kg body weight in men	
	14-22 mg/kg body weight in women	

12. After the physician has signed the Nutritional Assessment General Orders (Fig. 3), a nutrition technician from the Department of

(p. 29)

Dietetics Nutritional Assessment Program is authorized to verbal order times and dates for standard laboratory testing at ten-day intervals in the physicians order section of the Medical Record. Serial laboratory tests are ordered in this manner on the day prior to actual collection to allow adequate time for the physician to sign the orders.

13. All laboratory testing for nutritional assessment purposes is ordered on specific Nutritional Assessment Laboratory Requisitions (Fig. 19). These five-part forms are utilized so that an extra copy is available for delivery to the Nutritional Assessment Center to facilitate rapid communication of test results.

14. Collection of the 24-hour urine sample for urinary creatinine and urea nitrogen results is the responsibility of the staff nurse and coordination of the urine collection is the responsibility of the nurse in charge (see Section II-M).

15. All blood samples will be drawn by a trained technician from the Department of Pathology. Blood and urine samples will be delivered to the appropriate laboratories by this technician.

16. All laboratory testing is supervised by a medical technologist.

17. The results of laboratory tests ordered for nutritional assessment purposes will be delivered directly to the Nutritional Assessment center by a laboratory clerk on a daily basis.

EQUIPMENT

- Three Department of Pathology Chemistry Nutritional Assessment Laboratory requisitions (Fig. 19)
- One Department of Pathology Hematology Nutritional Assessment Laboratory Requisition
- Black ballpoint pen
- Red pen
- Medical record
- Addressograph

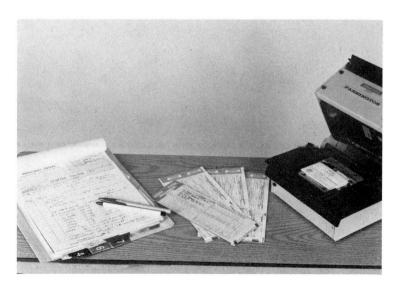

PROCEDURE

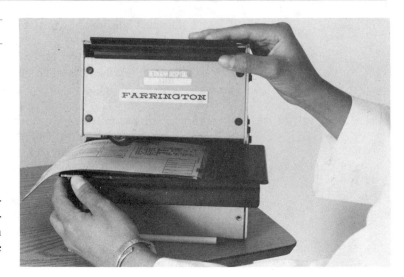

1. Stamp each Nutritional Assessment Laboratory requisition with the addressograph and check to ensure that the imprint is legible.

2. Complete a separate requisition for each laboratory of the Department of Pathology that will process test results, i.e.:

   a. (Blood chemistry) serum albumin, serum osmolarity.

   b. (Immunology) serum transferrin, prealbumin and/or retinol-binding protein.

   c. (Urine chemistry) 24-hour urine urea nitrogen, 24-hour urine creatinine.

   d. (Hematology) white blood cell count (WBC), differential for lymphocytes.

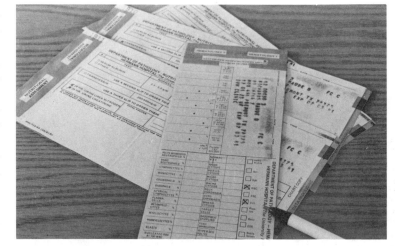

3. Using a red pen, order the 24-hour urine collection in the Physician's Order section of the medical record. Specify times and dates of specimen collection.

Sign the name of the physician that signed the Nutritional Assessment General Orders as a verbal order (V.O.) followed by the name of the dietitian with the technician's initials in parentheses.

Order the remaining laboratory testing in the same manner; specify date for actual collection.

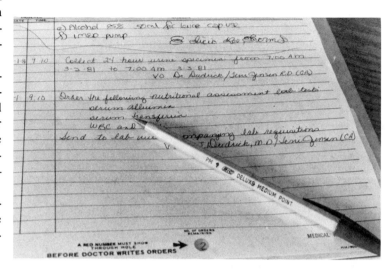

4. Fold the page with these new orders and attached laboratory requisitions with a paper clip. Return chart to the ward clerk to ensure that orders are communicated appropriately.

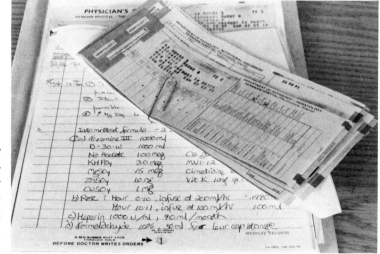

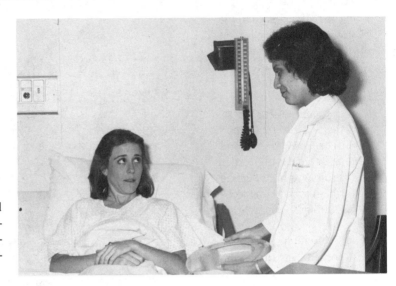

5. Instruct primary nurse and patient on the correct procedure for collecting the 24-hour urine sample (see Section II-M).

PATIENT TEACHING

1. Ensure that patient understands the purpose of laboratory testing.
2. Ensure that patient understands the procedure for collecting the 24-hour urine sample.

REFERENCES

1. Bistrian, B.R.: Therapeutic index of nutritional depletion in hospitalized patients. Surg. Gynecol. Obstet. 141:152, 1975.
2. Mackenzie, T., et al.: Clinical assessment of nutritional status using nitrogen balance. Fed. Proc. 33:683, 1947.
3. Rowlands, B.J., Jensen, T.G., Dudrick, S.J.: Serum transferrin—a comparison of two methods for measuring in hospitalized patients. Am. J. Clin. Nutr. 32:XIX, 1979.
4. Saubulich, H., et al.: Laboratory Test for the Assessment of Nutritional Status. Cleveland: CRC Press, 1974.
5. Viteri, F. and Alvarado, J.: The creatinine height index: Its use in the estimation of the degree of protein depletion and repletion in protein calorie malnourished children. Pediatrics 46:696, 1979.

M. Procedure for Collection of 24-Hour Urine Specimen _____

PURPOSE

The purposes of the procedure for collection of 24-hour urine specimen are:

1. To collect a urine specimen that represents the entire urinary output of a patient over a 24-hour period for quantitative, analytic, laboratory testing.
2. To ensure that the patient understands the procedure and cooperates during the collection period.

GENERAL INFORMATION

1. When an accumulated urine specimen is ordered, all urine voided for exactly 24 hours is measured.
2. Collection of the 24-hour urine specimen is the responsibility of the staff nurse. Supervision and coordination of the urine collection is the responsibility of the charge nurse.
3. The 24-hour urine collection is an important component of the Nutritional Assessment Program. The 24-hour specimen is analyzed for determination of urea nitrogen which is used to calculate nitrogen balance and creatinine excretion to indicate skeletal muscle protein catabolism.
4. Nitrogen balance compares nitrogen ingested with nitrogen excreted in the urine for an estimation of nitrogen retention. Therefore, if the urine is being collected for quantitation of urea nitrogen, simultaneous records of all oral, enteral and/or parenteral nutrient intake must also be recorded during the collection period.
5. A successful collection requires complete understanding and cooperation from the patient and all nursing personnel involved in the patient's care during the collection period.
6. The female patient must understand that separate bedpans must be used for urination and defecation during the collection period.

Toilet paper must not be discarded in the bedpan used for urine collection.

7. It is important to measure and record the amount of urine collected following each voiding, since the total volume of urine must be determined at the end of the collection period.

8. A cool storage temperature is required to prevent deterioration of the urine specimen and the sample should be stored in an ice bath during the collection period.

EQUIPMENT

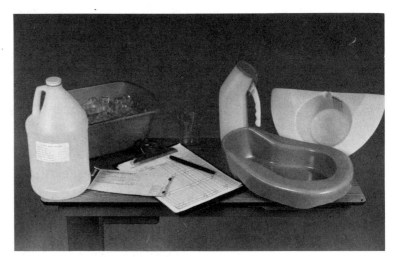

- One gallon specimen container
- Label for container
- Laboratory requisition
- Graduate for measuring and pouring
- Bedpan, urinal and cover or specimen collection unit
- Ice bath
- Pen or pencil

PROCEDURE

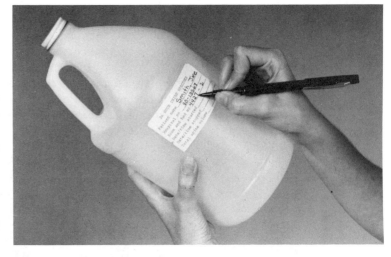

1. Label the one-gallon specimen container with the following information:
   a. 24-hour urine specimen label.
   b. Patient's full name.
   c. Patient's hospital number.
   d. Patient's room number and bed number.

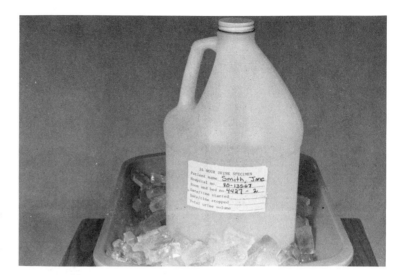

2. Store the container in an ice bath in a designated area, away from the patient's room.

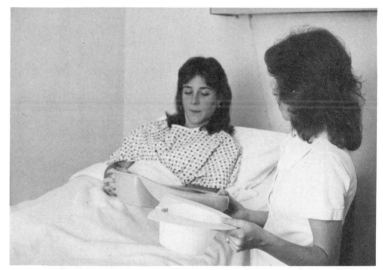

3. Identify patient and explain that all voided urine is measured and saved during the 24-hour collection period. Ensure that the patient understands the entire procedure.

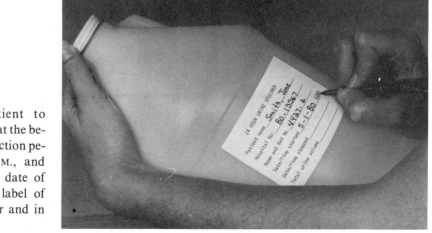

4. Instruct the patient to empty the bladder at the beginning of the collection period, i.e., 7:00 A.M., and note the time and date of this first void on label of specimen container and in the nurse's notes.

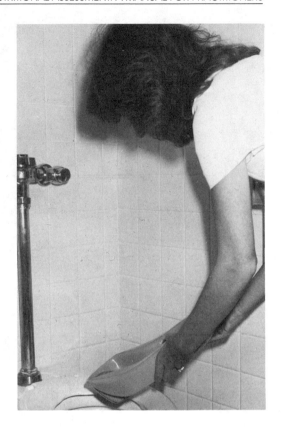

5. Discard this specimen.

6. Collect and save all urine voided during the 24-hour period after the first voiding. Each time the patient voids, pour the urine from the bedpan or urinal into the graduate to determine the volume of urine collected.

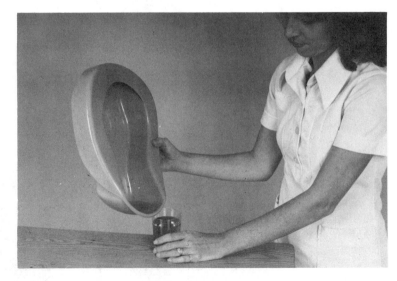

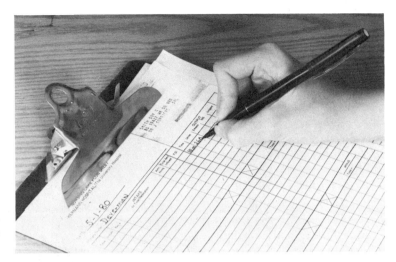

7. Record the amount voided on intake and output records.

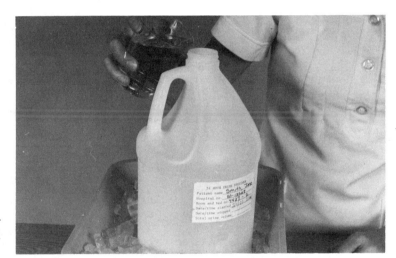

8. Pour the urine into the specimen container and store all collected urine on ice.

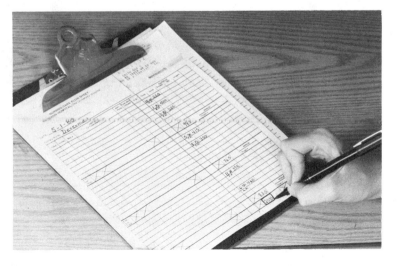

9. At the end of 24 hours , at the same hour, i.e., 7:00 A.M., that the collection period started, ask patient to void. Measure and record the amount and pour into specimen container. This is the end of the collection. Total the number of cc added to the specimen container and record this total and the time and date that the collection period ended on the container label.

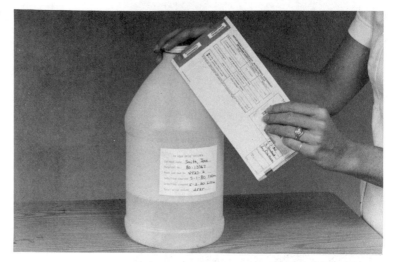

10. Secure the top of the container and attach the laboratory requisition. If the 24-hour urine is collected as part of the nutritional assessment procedure, the blue nutritional assessment laboratory requisition must be attached.

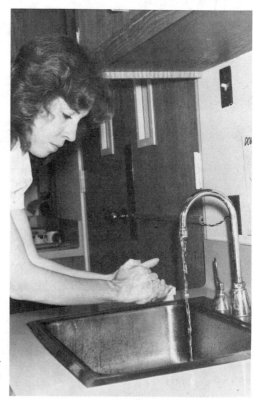

11. Wash hands. Enter the sample on the laboratory collection log. Send or take the labeled specimen with the requisition to the laboratory.

RECORDING AND REPORTING

1. Chart the procedure—the time and dates of specimen collection, the total volume of urine collected and sent to the lab—in nurse's notes.
2. Chart any collection error or other pertinent data which might influence the validity of the test in any manner, i.e., occurrence of menstruation, diarrhea, vaginal discharge, etc.

3. Chart any unusual observations concerning color, odor or consistency of urine.

REFERENCES

1. Hornemann, G.V.: Collection of specimens urine, in Basic Nursing Procedures. Albany, New York: Delmar Publications, 1972, pp. 69-72.
2. Leake, M.J.: Collecting a specimen of urine, in A Manual of Simple Nursing Procedures. Philadelphia: W.B. Saunders, 1971, pp. 74-75.
3. Ohio Trade and Industrial Education Service: Specimens, collection of urine, in Nursing Procedures for the Practical Nurse. State Department of Education, 1972, pp. 227-231.

N. Procedure for Transferring Skin Test Antigen Solutions from Vials to Syringes _____

The purposes of the procedure for transferring skin test antigen solutions from vials to syringes are:

1. To prepare syringes for injection of skin test antigen solutions.
2. To ensure accurate dosages of skin test antigen preparations.
3. To ensure accurate labeling of skin test syringes.
4. To ensure patient safety.

GENERAL INFORMATION

1. Skin antigen testing is an integral component of the comprehensive nutritional assessment procedure.
2. Skin testing detects cutaneous hypersensitivity to one or a group of antigens and is used to assess immunocompetence and visceral protein status. Since most of the population has had contact or infection with the various agents, a delayed cutaneous hypersensitivity response is usually demonstrated if the immune system is intact.
3. Four skin test antigens are applied for nutritional assessment purposes at Hermann Hospital. The following antigens are routinely administered*:

Antigen	Supplier
Trichophyton Mix 1000 PNU/ml	Hollister-Stier, Dallas, TX 75234
Candida (monilia) Albicans 1000 PNU/ml	Lederle Laboratories, Pearl River, NY 1096
Mumps Skin Test Antigen	Eli Lilly and Co., Indianapolis, IN 46206

* Streptokinase-Streptodornase (SK-SD) Varidase is also applied when available from the manufacturer, Lederle Laboratories, Pearl River, NY 10965.

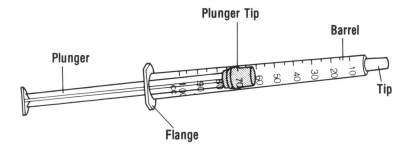

Figure 20. Tuberculin Syringe. A 0.1 ml tuberculin syringe is used to apply skin test antigens.

Antigen	Supplier
Tuberculin Purified Protein Derivative, Aplisol®, diluted 5 IU/0.1 ml	Park Davis and Co., Detroit, MI 48232

4. The administration of skin test antigen preparations requires transfer of solutions from vials to syringes. Careful adherence to defined procedure is essential to ensure patient safety.

5. Skin test antigen solutions are transferred from vials to syringes by nutrition support nurses on the day before they are to be administered.

6. The vial is a sterile glass container. Every vial has a rubber diaphragm covering which protects the sterility of the solution contained in the vial. The rubber diaphragm is penetrated by a needle in order to transfer solution from the vial into the syringe. Despite the metal cap or flip-top cap which covers the diaphragm, it is never considered sterile; therefore, the rubber diaphragm surface must always be cleansed with an alcohol pledget before the needle is inserted into the diaphragm.

7. Prior to transferring solution from a vial into a syringe, one should inspect the vial. The vial must never be used when (1) the glass is broken; (2) the solution is cloudy; or (3) particles are found inside the vial.

8. The disposable syringe consists of five parts (Fig. 20):
   a. Barrel: The barrel of the syringe contains graduated markings in cc to measure the proper amounts of solution to be drawn from the vial.
   b. Tip: The tip of the syringe is inserted into the needle hub.
   c. Flange: The rim of the barrel at the end opposite the tip prevents the syringe from rolling when it is placed on a flat surface.
   d. Plunger: The plunger is a movable cylinder that slides in and out of the barrel as the solution is transferred into and out of the syringe.
   e. Plunger tip: The position of the plunger tip along the graduated markings on the barrel is a measurement of the amount of solution or air in the syringe.

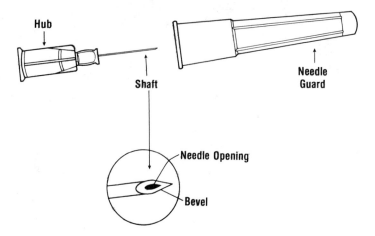

Figure 21. Needle. A short beveled (3/8-5/8 inch), 27 gauge needle is attached to the tuberculin syringe for the intradermal injection of skin test antigens.

9. The disposable needle consists of five parts (Fig. 21):
   a. Hub: The tip of the syringe is inserted into the hub of the needle.
   b. Bevel: The point or bevel of the needle is sharp so that it can be used for penetration of the rubber diaphragm or body tissue when administering medication or solutions intramuscularly, intradermally or subcutaneously.
   c. Needle opening: The gauge of the needle is determined by the diameter of the needle opening. As the gauge of the needle increases, the diameter of the needle opening decreases, and vice versa. Thus, a needle with a gauge of 27 has smaller needle opening than a needle with a gauge of 16.
   d. Shaft: The shaft is the length of the needle and varies according to the type of injection administered, i.e., catheter irrigation, intramuscular injection or subcutaneous injection. Short needle shafts are used for intradermal injections.
   e. Needle guard: The needle guard protects the sterility of the needle when it is not being used.
10. Contamination of the solution during the transfer from vial to syringe can result in infection. Contaminants from the hands must be removed by proper handwashing technique to minimize the possibility of infection.
11. The needle must be inserted into the vial as outlined in this procedure to prevent pieces of the rubber diaphragm from "breaking off" into the solution as the needle repeatedly penetrates the rubber diaphragm.
12. Air is injected into the vial prior to transferring the solution because failure to inject air would create a partial vacuum, thereby making it difficult to remove solution from the vial. The amount of air injected is equal to the solution to be withdrawn from the vial.

13. Air bubbles must be removed from the syringe by tapping the syringe lightly with fingertips to ensure that the proper amount of solution is contained in the syringe.
14. Skin test antigens are administered by a nutrition support nurse and responses are read at 24 and 48 hours following injection by the same nurse (see Sections II-O and II-P).

EQUIPMENT

- 4 disposable 1 ml tuberculin syringes with 27 gauge, 1/2 inch detachable needles
- Alcohol pledgets
- Vial(s) Trichophyton Mix 1000 PNU/ml
- Vial(s) Candida (monilia) Albicans 1000 PNU/ml
- Vial(s) mumps skin test antigen
- Vial(s) Tuberculin PPD, Aplisol® 5 TU/0.1 ml
- Black pen

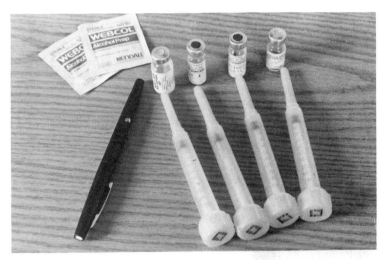

PROCEDURE

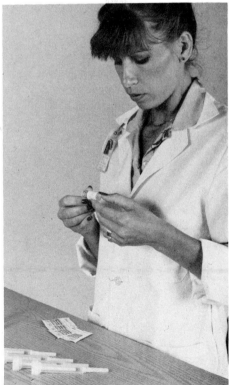

1. Determine number of injections to be prepared and assemble equipment accordingly. Check the expiration date on each vial.

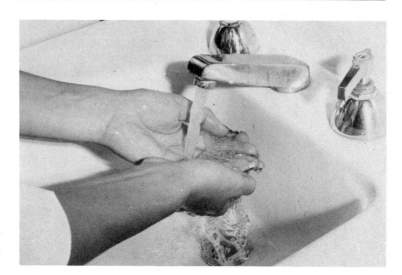

2. Wash hands using the recommended handwashing technique.

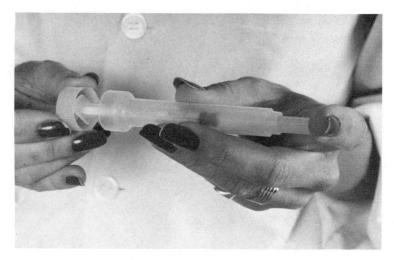

3. Remove the plastic covering from the syringe by twisting the cap away from the syringe and pushing the needle guard toward the covering with the forefinger of the opposite hand. Discard both plastic pieces in the waste container.

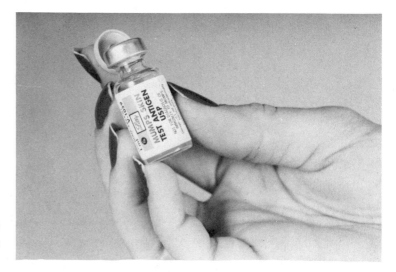

4. Remove the cap from the antigen vial and discard in the trash container.

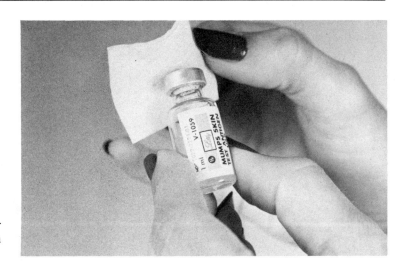

5. Cleanse the rubber diaphragm of the vial with an antiseptic alcohol pad.

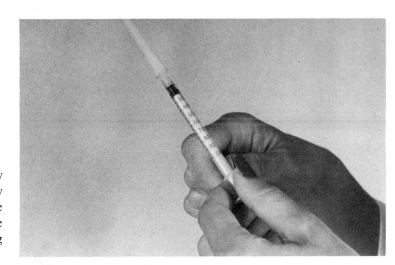

6. Draw air into the syringe by moving the plunger away from the needle until the plunger tip is situated on the 0.1 ml graduated marking of the syringe.

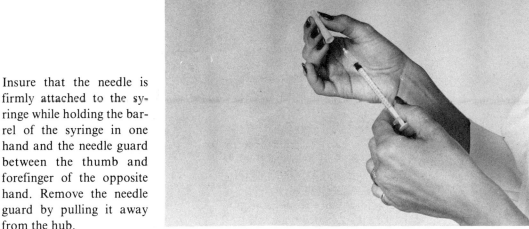

7. Insure that the needle is firmly attached to the syringe while holding the barrel of the syringe in one hand and the needle guard between the thumb and forefinger of the opposite hand. Remove the needle guard by pulling it away from the hub.

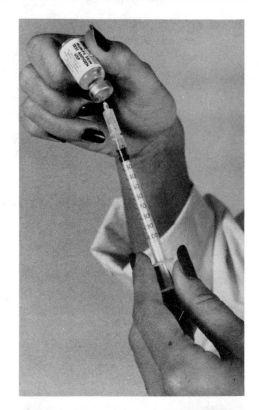

8. Without touching the rubber diaphragm, invert the vial and hold with the thumb, forefinger and palm of one hand. Insert the needle into the center of the rubber diaphragm at a 45° angle with the bevel side up.

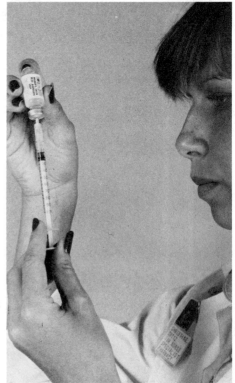

9. While holding the syringe perpendicular to the floor, inject 0.1 ml of air into the vial by depressing the plunger. Hold the needle perpendicular to the floor at eye level, with the bevel in solution and withdraw a little over 0.1 ml of the antigen preparation by pulling the plunger away from the needle until the plunger tip is situated just above the 0.1 ml graduated marking.

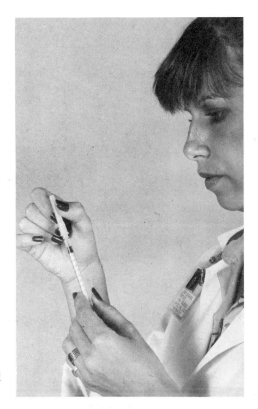

10. Withdraw the needle from the rubber diaphragm and replace the needle guard over the needle.

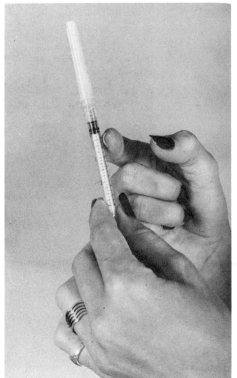

11. While holding the needle pointed toward the ceiling, remove any air bubbles by tapping the barrel of the syringe lightly with the fingertips until they disappear. Move the plunger gently toward the needle until the air is expelled from the syringe and 0.1 ml of solution remains in the syringe.

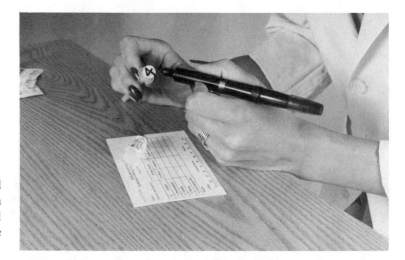

12. Check the label on the vial with the antigen number on the skin test data card and label the syringe with the correct antigen number.

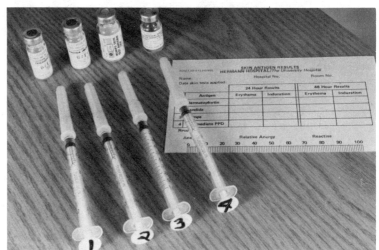

13. Repeat procedures 3 through 13 until all syringes are prepared and labeled for skin testing on the following day. Prepare all syringes with one antigen before transferring the other antigens from vials to syringes. Discard empty vials and store partially used multidose vials according to manufacturer's directions.

REFERENCES

1. Leake, M.J.: Procedure for preparing the injection, in A Manual of Simple Nursing Procedures. Philadelphia: W.B. Saunders, 1971, pp. 203-205.
2. Sorensen, K. and Luckman, K.C.: Preparing medications for injection and caring for equipment, in Basic Nursing: A Psychologist Approach. Philadelphia: W.B. Saunders, 1979, pp. 950-955.

O. Procedure for Intradermal Injection of Skin Test Antigens _____

The purposes of the procedure for intradermal injection of skin test antigens are:

1. To assess visceral protein status and cell-mediated immunity.
2. To identify pre- and postoperative patients at increased risk for sepsis and mortality.
3. To evaluate changes in skin reactivity at serial intervals during nutritional support.

1. Skin antigen testing is an integral component of the comprehensive nutritional assessment procedure. The increases in sepsis and mortality in patients with anergic skin test responses are highly significant, and patients with questionable nutritional status as indicated by screening assessment should be skin tested preoperatively whenever feasible or practical.
2. Skin test antigen preparations are administered by a nutrition support nurse and responses are read at 24 and 48 hours postinjection by the same nurse.
3. Because stress may obliterate the local reaction, skin test antigens should not be applied during the first 48 hours following major surgery or the first four to five days following severe thermal injury or multiple trauma.
4. Prior to the injection of skin test antigens, the patient should be questioned regarding results of any prior skin tests and allergies to any of the constituents of antigen preparations. Mumps skin test antigen is prepared from virus cultivated in chicken embryo and persons who are sensitive to an avian protein may have a severe reaction following administration of the antigen. Therefore, those

135

patients known to be sensitive to chicken, eggs or feathers should not be skin tested with mumps antigen. Pseudopositive reactions may also develop in patients sensitive to egg protein. Tuberculin PPD should not be administered to known tuberculin positive reactors since a severe reaction—vesiculation, ulceration, necrosis—may occur at the site in highly sensitized individuals.

5. A brief history of recent immunization and medications must also be ascertained. Reactivity to skin test antigens may be depressed or suppressed for as long as four to six weeks in individuals receiving concurrent or recent immunization with certain viral vaccines—measles, influenza, those who have had recent viral infections—rubeola, influenza, mumps, and those who are receiving corticosteroids or other immunosuppressive agents. All subjective data regarding skin antigen testing is recorded on the back of the Skin Test Data Card (Fig. 22).

6. The skin area selected for intradermal injections should be free of disease, i.e., psoriasis or eczema, which could be exacerbated or spread by injecting the antigen intradermally.

7. Also, avoid injecting skin test antigens into areas which may alter interpretation of local tissue responses such as:
   a. Areas that have previous irritation, discoloration, or swelling of the skin, scarring or pustular eruptions.
   b. Sites which could be irritated by clothing.

8. The preferred site for injection of skin test antigens is the volar aspect of the forearm. When this site is selected, the right and left arm should be alternated subsequently for serial testing.

9. Injury to the forearm may necessitate selection of an alternate skin area. Other preferential sites include:
   a. The right or left anterior upper thigh.
   b. Infrascapular thoracic back.
   c. Suprapubic anterior abdomen.

10. The series of antigens should always be injected in the same order—as specified on the Skin Test Data card—to avoid confusion in reading results.

11. The antigen injection site must be observed immediately after injection for the appearance of a wheal—small circular bump which appears whitened. The immediate appearance of a flat area with flat pseudopods radiating out indicates that air was present in the syringe. If no wheal is formed, the injection was subcutaneous rather than intracutaneous and must be repeated at another site. A strong immediate reaction at the injection site may result in a false negative delayed reaction and must be noted on the data card.

12. Rarely patients who are very sensitive to a particular antigen will have a severe local reaction at the injection site, which may include tissue necrosis, ulceration or vesiculation. Scar formation and/or hyperpigmentation may result with or without associated epitroclear or axillary adenopathy. Systemic effects, including fever and tachycardia, may occur very rarely.

EQUIPMENT

- Adhesive tape
- Five povidone-iodine pledgets
- Five 70 percent alcohol pledgets
- Four labeled tuberculin syringes with 26-27 gauge needle and short bevel (3/8 to 5/8 inch). Each syringe should contain 0.1 ml of one of the following antigens: Dermatophytin, Candida®, Mumps and Purified Protein Derivative
- Indelible marking pen
- Skin Test Data Card

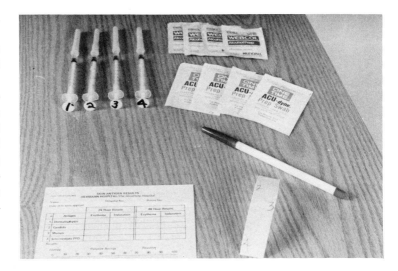

PROCEDURE

1. Identify the patient and ensure that he or she understands the procedure. Question the patient regarding results of previous skin test, the occurrence of severe reactions and allergies to chicken, eggs or feathers. Record any significant subjective information on the back of the Skin Test Data Card and select antigens accordingly. Also review current medications and recent immunizations and illnesses which would affect skin test results with the patient and record on the Skin Test Data Card (Fig. 22).

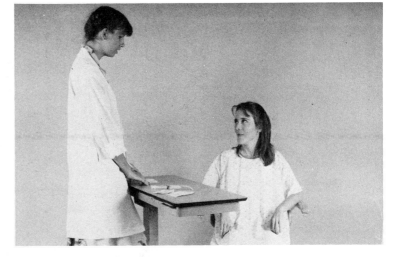

HH/730-37(10/80)

SKIN ANTIGEN RESULTS
HERMANN HOSPITAL/*The University Hospital*

Name: Hospital No.   Room No.

Date skin tests applied:

#	Antigen	24 Hour Results		48 Hour Results	
		Erythema	Induration	Erythema	Induration
1	Dermatophytin				
2	Candida				
3	Mumps				
4	Intermediate PPD				

Results:

Anergy   Relative Anergy   Reactive

0   10   20   30   40   50   60   70   80   90   100
|||||||||||||||||||||||||||||||||||||||||||||||||||||||||||||||||||||||||||||||||||||||||

Figure 22. Skin Test Data Card. Measurable erythema and induration are recorded on the skin test data card at 24 and 48 hours following the injection of antigens.

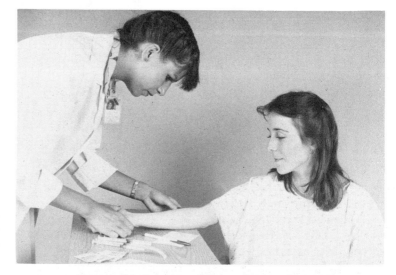

2. Assess condition of the skin and surrounding tissue. Select skin area where antigens will be injected.

3. Apply approximately 25 centimeters of tape to the skin area where antigens are to be injected. The skin test antigens must be applied at least 5 centimeters apart to prevent possible overlap of reactions. Label the tape with antigen numbers corresponding to those on the Skin Test Data Card (Fig. 22).

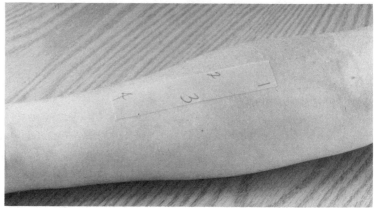

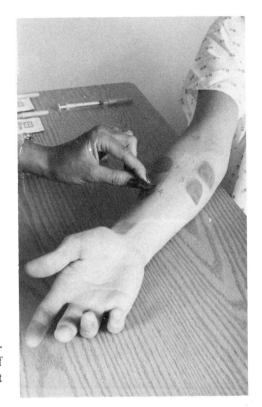

4. Vigorously cleanse the selected area with a povidone-iodine pledget, being careful not to touch the edges of the applied tape. Use a circular motion, starting at each injection site and moving outwards.

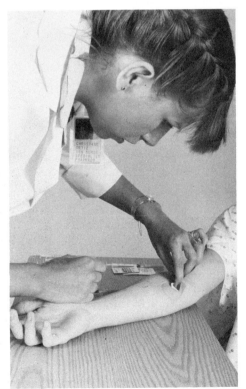

5. Remove povidone-iodine solution using a 70 percent alcohol pledget. Allow to dry.

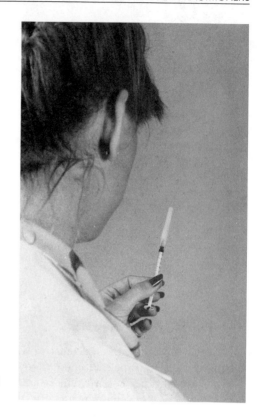

6. Check to ensure that each syringe contains only 0.1 ml of antigen.

7. Position the patient with his arm in a relaxed position, with the inner aspect of the arm exposed and elbow fixed. Grasp the middle of the patient's forearm, pulling the anterior skin taut. If skin tests are applied to a site other than the forearm, maneuver the skin until it can be pulled taut.

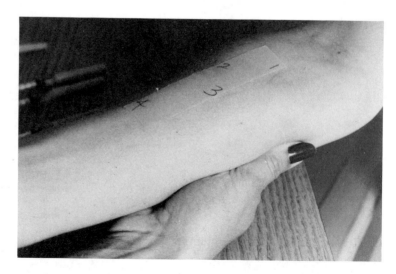

8. Holding the skin taut, insert the needle with the bevel up, to a depth of about 1/8 inch at an angle that allows the needle to enter between layers of skin (10 to 15 degrees to the skin). Check to ensure that the bevel is entirely covered by the skin. The bevel should be visible through the skin when the injection is properly administered.

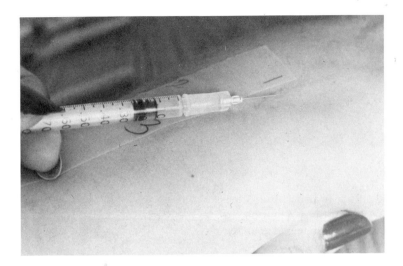

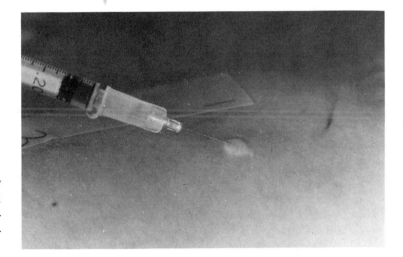

9. Inject the antigen slowly by depressing the plunger and observe the patient carefully for any unusual reaction.

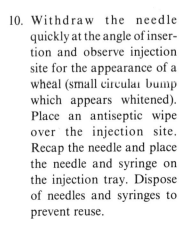

10. Withdraw the needle quickly at the angle of insertion and observe injection site for the appearance of a wheal (small circular bump which appears whitened). Place an antiseptic wipe over the injection site. Recap the needle and place the needle and syringe on the injection tray. Dispose of needles and syringes to prevent reuse.

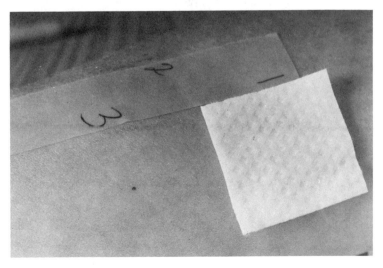

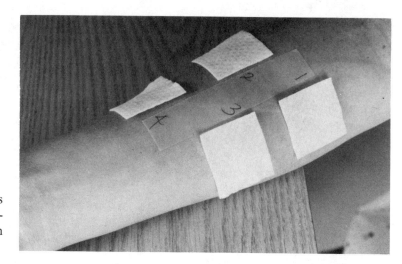

11. Repeat procedural steps 1-10 with each antigen, applying antigens at least 5 cm apart.

12. Complete the following information on the Skin Test Data Card and return the card to the Nutritional Assessment Center:

   a. Patient's name.
   b. Room number.
   c. Hospital number.
   d. Date and time of application of skin test.
   e. Location of application.

REPORTING AND RECORDING

1. Chart that skin test antigens have been applied in the progress notes of the medical record, note the antigens used, location of application, date and time of application and time when reactions are to be read.

2. Any unusual reaction such as immediate respiratory rate increase, wheezing, tachycardia, itching and/or rash must be reported immediately to the physician.

3. Complete the Skin Test Data Card and return it to the nutritional assessment center.

REFERENCES

1. Bonewit, K.: Administration of medications, in Clinical Procedures for Medical Assistants. Philadelphia: W.B. Saunders, 1979, pp. 205-206.

2. Copeland, E.M., MacFadyen, B.V. Jr., and Dudrick, S.J.: Effect of intra-

venous hyperalimentation on established delayed hypersensitivity in cancer patients. Ann. Surg. 184:61, 1976.

3. Law, D.K., Dudrick, S.J., and Abdou, N.I.: Immunocompetence of patients with protein-calorie malnutrition. Ann. Int. Med. 79:545, 1973.

4. Meakins, J.L., Pietsch, J.B., et al.: Delayed hypersensitivity: Indicator of acquired failure of host defenses in sepsis and trauma. Ann. Surg. 186:241, 1977.

5. Sokal, J.E.: Measurement of delayed skin test response. N. Engl. J. Med. 501, 1975.

6. Sorenson, K. and Luckman, K.C.: Intradermal and subcutaneous injection, in Basic Nursing. A Physiological Approach. Philadelphia: W.B. Saunders, 1979, pp. 974-980.

P. Procedure for Measuring and Interpreting Skin Test Reactions _____

The purposes of the procedure for measuring and interpreting skin test reactions are:

1. To assess visceral protein status and cell-mediated immunity.
2. To identify pre- and postoperative patients at increased risk for sepsis and related mortality.
3. To evaluate restoration of skin reactivity at ten-day intervals during nutritional support.

1. Skin antigen testing is an integral component of the comprehensive nutritional assessment procedure.
2. Skin test reactions are read and interpreted at 24 and 48 hours following injection by the nutrition support nurse that administered the skin test antigens.
3. Reactions are interpreted from measurements of induration at 24 and/or 48 hours. A reactive response is defined as induration greater than or equal to 5 mm to any one antigen at 24 and/or 48 hours. An indurated response of 1-4 mm is considered relative anergy and no measurable induration at either time denotes anergy.
4. When anergic or relatively anergic reactions are noted, skin testing is continued as part of the serial nutritional assessment at ten-day intervals until restoration of reactivity is achieved.
5. When a patient responds to a particular antigen with induration greater than 30 millimeters, the serial skin test procedure for that antigen is discontinued to avoid the possibility of a severe local reaction.

EQUIPMENT

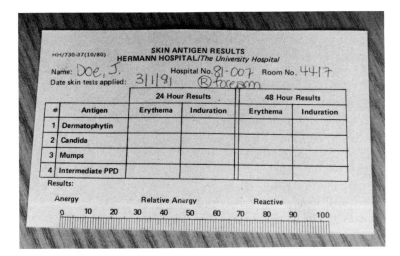

- Ball point pen (medium point)
- Skin Test Data Card

PROCEDURE

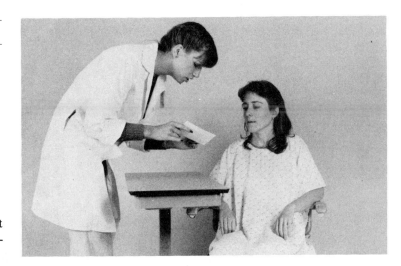

1. Explain procedure to patient and ensure that he or she understands procedure.

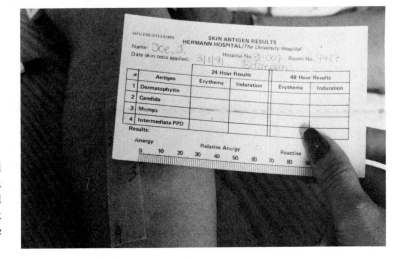

2. Measure the length and width of the area of erythema (pinkness or redness) around each antigen injection site at 24 hours with the ruled edge of the skin test card.

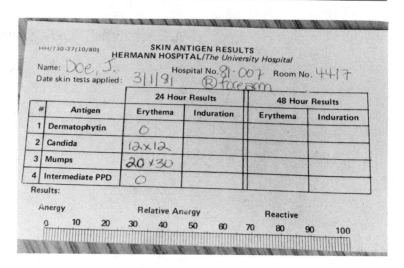

3. Record the length by the width of the erythematous area on the Skin Test Data Card in the appropriate space at 24 hours. If no erythema is observed at any one or all of the skin test sites, record a "0" in the appropriate space (Fig. 22).

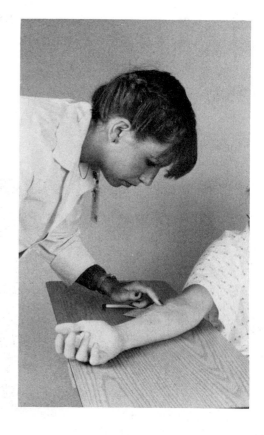

4. Carefully palpate each injection site for a firm mass.

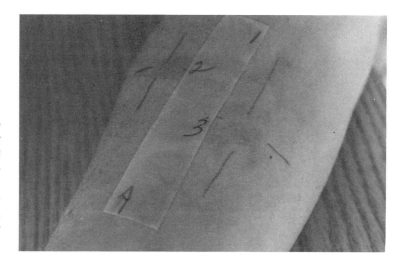

5. If induration is detected, mark the margin of induration by lightly moving the ball point pen toward the injection site from four sides. Definite resistance to further movement is noted when the pen reaches the margin of induration.

Name: Doe, J.　Hospital No. 81-007　Room No. 441				
Date skin tests applied: 3/1/81　Ⓡ forearm				
		24 Hour Results		48 Hour Results
#	Antigen	Erythema	Induration	Erythema	Indura
1	Dermatophytin	O			
2	Candida	12×12			
3	Mumps	20×30			
4	Intermediate PPD	O			

Results:

Anergy　　　Relative Anergy　　　Reactive
0　10　20　30　40　50　60　70　80　90　100

6. Measure the length and width of the marked induration with the ruled edge of the Skin Test Data Card.

HH/730-37(10/80)

SKIN ANTIGEN RESULTS
HERMANN HOSPITAL/*The University Hospital*

Name: Doe, J.　　Hospital No. 81-007　Room No. 4417				
Date skin tests applied: 3/1/81　Ⓡ forearm				
		24 Hour Results		48 Hour Results	
#	Antigen	Erythema	Induration	Erythema	Induration
1	Dermatophytin	Ө	Ө		
2	Candida	12×12	7×10		
3	Mumps	20×30	15×15		
4	Intermediate PPD	Ө	Ө		

Results:

Anergy　　　Relative Anergy　　　Reactive
0　10　20　30　40　50　60　70　80　90　100

7. Record measurements of induration in the appropriate space on the Skin Test Data Card and in the progress notes of the medical record.

8. Repeat steps 2 through 7 again at 48 hours following injection. Instruct the patient to report any increase in the reaction occurring after 48 hours.

9. Interpret skin test results according to the largest measured area of induration (length or width) at 24 and/ or 48 hours. Circle the interpretation on the Skin Test Data Card.

REPORTING AND RECORDING

1. Record measured erythema and induration at 24 and 48 hours in the progress notes of the medical record and on the Skin Test Data Card.

2. Record the interpretation of the reaction in the progress notes of the medical record and on the Skin Test Data Card.

3. Report any unusual reaction or response to the physician immediately.

4. Discontinue serial skin testing, when any response to a particular antigen exceeds 30 millimeters induration.

5. Return the completed Skin Test Data Card to the Nutritional Assessment Center.

REFERENCE

1. Sokal, J.E.: Measurement of delayed skin test response. N. Engl. J. Med. 501, 1975.

Section III
Guidelines for Interpreting Nutritional Assessment Data

A. Weight/Height

In addition to precise and accurate data collection, the cautious interpretation of assimilated objective nutritional assessment data is imperative to classify the type of malnutrition and to estimate the magnitude of nutritional depletion in a given case. The therapeutic support regimen in each case can be effectively formulated and evaluated only through such careful data interpretation. This section summarizes the clinical significance, calculations, standards, and normal ranges and the clinical considerations for accurate interpretation of objective measurements and tests in current use for the nutritional assessment of hospitalized patients.

CLINICAL SIGNIFICANCE

Body weight is the most accessible and widely used index of nutritional status in hospitalized patients. As a simple measure of gross body composition, the body weight is a valuable screening indicator of nutritional risk when compared with the patient's usual weight, desirable weight, or both. Additionally, weight change is an important indicator of nutritional rehabilitation when measured regularly and accurately and in conjunction with a significant knowledge of relevant clinical and biochemical variables. Weight changes can be calculated as percentages of the patient's usual weight, admission weight, pretherapy weight, or last-assessment weight to provide clinically valuable information.

Several surveys have verified that a significant proportion of hospitalized patients report recent weight loss or are below a desirable weight for their height.[1-3] Generally, an unintentional weight loss of greater than 10 pounds within a 6-month period is considered significant.[4] A history of weight loss and/or a weight for height that is less than 85 percent of the desirable weight have been related to functional consequences and complications of malnutrition.[4,5] Additionally, a significant increase in mortality has been positively correlated with a history of weight loss.[6] Seltzer et al. have correlated an absolute weight loss of more than 10 pounds with a 19-fold increase in mortality in 4382 elective adult surgical patients.[7]

CALCULATIONS

Calculations for interpreting weight change and weight-for-height changes include:

$$\% \text{ Desirable weight} = \frac{\text{Present weight}}{\text{Desirable weight}} \times 100$$

$$\% \text{ Usual weight} = \frac{\text{Present weight}}{\text{Usual weight}} \times 100$$

$$\% \text{ Weight change (usual weight)} = \frac{\text{Usual weight} - \text{Present weight}}{\text{Usual weight}} \times 100$$

$$\% \text{ Weight change (admission weight)} = \frac{\text{Admission weight} - \text{Present weight}}{\text{Admission weight}} \times 100$$

$$\% \text{ Weight change (pretherapy)} = \frac{\text{Pretherapy weight} - \text{Present weight}}{\text{Pretherapy weight}} \times 100$$

$$\% \text{ Weight change (since last assessment)} = \frac{\text{Last weight} - \text{Present weight}}{\text{Last weight}} \times 100$$

STANDARDS

Data from the Health and Nutrition Examination Survey and the Metropolitan Life Insurance company are the primary sources used in evaluating weight-for-height measurements.[8,9] Considerable controversy has arisen over the appropriateness of these standards for evaluating measurements in hospitalized patients.[5,10,11] The Metropolitan Life Insurance standards are based on measurements taken on men and women insured by a number of life insurance companies in the United States and Canada between 1935 and 1954. The measurements were taken on subjects wearing shoes and clothing, and have been adapted to nude weights by subtracting a fixed amount from the weight to represent clothing, and to heights without shoe heels by subtracting a fixed amount from the height to compensate for the heel height (Table 1).[12,13] The validity of these corrections is questionable because of the variability in clothing weights and shoe heels in the original study. Nevertheless, the Metropolitan Life Insurance standards have been used historically to diagnose obesity, and have been related to mortality in hospitalized patients.[5]

Desirable weights can also be ascertained from the Health and Nutrition Examination Survey, which is a probability sample of 28,000 noninstitutionalized Americans conducted from 1971 to 1974 (Table 2). All subjects in this study were measured without shoes; their cloth-

TABLE 1. IDEAL WEIGHT FOR HEIGHT   *Old Data*

Males				Females			
Height (cm)	Weight (kg)	Height (cm)	Weight (kg)	Height (cm)	Weight (kg)	Height (cm)	Weight (kg)
145	51.9	166	64.0	140	44.9	155	53.1
146	52.4	167	64.6	141	45.4	156	53.7
147	52.9	168	65.2	142	45.9	157	54.3
148	53.5	169	65.9	143	46.4	158	54.9
149	54.0	170	66.6	144	47.0	159	55.5
150	54.5	171	67.3	145	47.5	160	56.2
151	55.0	172	68.0	146	48.0	161	56.9
152	55.6	173	68.7	147	48.6	162	57.6
153	56.1	174	69.4	148	49.2	163	58.3
154	56.6	175	70.1	149	49.8	164	58.9
155	57.2	176	70.8	150	50.4	165	59.5
156	57.9	177	71.6	151	51.0	166	60.1
157	58.6	178	72.4	152	51.5	167	60.7
158	59.3	179	73.3	153	52.0	168	61.4
159	59.9	180	74.2	154	52.5	169	62.1
160	60.5	181	75.0				
161	61.1	182	75.8				
162	61.7	183	76.5				
163	62.3	184	77.3				
164	62.9	185	78.1				
165	63.5	186	78.9				

This table corrects the 1959 Metropolitan Standards to nude weight without shoe heels. (From Blackburn CL, et al.: Nutritional and metabolic assessment of the hospitalized patient. J.P.E.N. 1:11–20, 1977, adapted from Jelliffe, D.B.: The Assessment of the Nutritional Status of the Community, W.H.O., Geneva, 1966.)

ing weights varied from 0.2 to 0.8 pounds. Data from this survey are also more current than those from the Metropolitan Life Insurance survey, and are therefore considered more representative of the American population.

DATA INTERPRETATION

An initial baseline body weight of less than 90 percent of the desirable weight for a given height, or less than 5 percent of the usual weight, or a recent unintentional weight loss of greater than 10 pounds is considered indicative of nutritional risk.[4,5] A weight loss of greater than 20 percent of the premorbid body weight indicates an increased mortality risk.[6] Although these calculations provide clinically significant information, caution is essential in their interpretation since some disease states are characterized by abnormalities in body composition. Ascites, pleural effusion, and anasarca may be accompanied by weight gain caused by an imbalance in the mechanisms that maintain intravascular and intracellular homeostasis. In the malnourished state, the expansion of extracellular fluid and simultaneous depletion of lean body mass lessen the reliability of weight as an indicator of nutritional status. However, in most instances, the initial body weight will provide an indication of the need for more comprehensive nutritional evaluation.

TABLE 2. IDEAL WEIGHT-FOR-HEIGHT ACCORDING TO AGE AND SEX*

Sex and Height	Ages					
	18–24	25–34	35–44	45–54	55–64	65–74
Men						
62 inches	130	141	143	147	143	143
63 inches	135	145	148	152	147	147
64 inches	140	150	153	156	153	151
65 inches	145	156	158	160	158	156
66 inches	150	160	163	164	163	160
67 inches	154	165	169	169	168	164
68 inches	159	170	174	173	173	169
69 inches	164	174	179	177	178	173
70 inches	168	179	184	182	183	177
71 inches	173	184	190	187	189	182
72 inches	178	189	194	191	193	186
73 inches	183	194	200	196	197	190
74 inches	188	199	205	200	203	194
Women						
57 inches	114	118	125	129	132	130
58 inches	117	121	129	133	136	134
59 inches	120	125	133	136	140	137
60 inches	123	128	137	140	143	140
61 inches	126	132	141	143	147	144
62 inches	129	136	144	147	150	147
63 inches	132	139	148	150	153	151
64 inches	135	142	152	154	157	154
65 inches	138	146	156	158	160	158
66 inches	141	150	159	161	164	161
67 inches	144	153	163	165	167	165
68 inches	147	157	167	168	171	169

*All heights were measured without shoes. The total weights of all clothing ranged from 0.20 to 0.62 pounds, which was not deducted from the weights shown. (Data obtained from the Health and Nutrition Examination Survey, 1971–1974.) (Adapted from Weight by Height and Age of Adults 18–74 Years: United States, 1971–1974. DHEW Publication No. (PHS) 79-1656, Series II, No. 208. Hyattsville, MD: U.S. Department of Health, Education, and Welfare, 1979, p. 34.)

In general, a 1/4- to 1/2-pound weight gain per day is indicative of a reasonable accumulation of lean body tissue in patients receiving hyperalimentation. A more rapid weight change of greater than 1 pound per day usually suggests fluid imbalance. However, the patient with severe protein depletion may experience a weight gain of 3 to 4 pounds during the first 48 to 72 hours of rehydration owing to expansion of extracellular fluid volume. The early postadmission weight of the multiple-trauma or thermally injured patient may be elevated 12 to 15 percent above the patient's usual pre-injury weight as a consequence of massive fluid resuscitation. In contrast, the cachectic patient with anasarca may lose body weight during the introduction of nutritional therapy in response to an increase in colloid osmotic pressure and subsequent diuresis.

REFERENCES

1. Hill, G.L., Blacket, R.L., Rickford, I., et al.: Malnutrition in surgical patients: An unrecognized problem. Lancet 1:689–692, 1977.
2. Bistrian, B.R., Blackburn, G.L., Vitale, J., et al.: Prevalence of malnutrition in general medical patients. JAMA 235:1567–1570, 1976.
3. Bistrian, B.R., Blackburn, G.L., Hallowell, E., et al.: Protein status of general surgical patients. JAMA 230:858–860, 1974.
4. Harvey, K.B., Riggiero, J.A., Regan, C.S., et al.: Hospital morbidity-mortality risk factors using nutritional assessment. Clin. Res. 26:581, 1978.
5. Bistrian, B.R.: Anthropometric norms used in assessment of hospitalized patients. Am. J. Clin. Nutr. 33:2211–2214, 1980.
6. Studley, H.O.: Percentage of weight loss—A basic indicator of surgical risk in patients with chronic peptic ulcer. JAMA 106:458, 1936.
7. Seltzer, M.H., Slocom, B.A., and Cataldi-Belcher, E.L.: Instant nutritional assessment: Absolute weight loss and surgical mortality. JPEN 6:218, 1982.
8. National Center for Health Statistics. Weight by Height and Age of Adults 18–74 years: United States, 1971–1974. Rockville, MD: National Center for Health Statistics, 1979. (Vital and Health Statistics. Series II: Data from the National Health Survey, No. 208) [DHEW publication No. (PHS) 79-1656].
9. Build and Blood Pressure Study. Chicago: Chicago Society of Actuaries, 1959.
10. Gray, G.E. and Gray, L.K.: Validity of anthropometric norms used in the assessment of hospitalized patients. JPEN 5:366–368, 1979.
11. Gray, G.E. and Gray, L.K.: Anthropometric measurements and their interpretation: principles, practices and problems. J. Am. Diet. Assoc. 77:534–539, 1980.
12. Grant, A.: Section B: Anthropometry. In Nutritional Assessment Guidelines, Distributed by Cutter Medical, 1979.
13. Blackburn, G.L., Bistrian, B.R., and Mani, B.S., et al.: Nutritional and metabolic assessment of the hospitalized patient. JPEN 1:11, 1979.

B. Upper Arm Anthropometry

Subcutaneous fat stores, evaluated by measurement of the triceps skinfold, play an insignificant role in daily body metabolism, but depletion of this compartment can reflect chronic energy deprivation. Similarly, skeletal muscle catabolism occurs following either protein or energy deprivation and may be detected by calculation of the arm muscle circumference and/or area. In the absence of an adequate exogenous supply of calories, energy is generated primarily by lipolysis and the conversion of tissue protein into glucose via gluconeogenesis, resulting in a reduction of adipose and somatic-tissue protein reserves. When the body's protein requirements are not met, amino acids are transported from skeletal muscle stores to the viscera to support liver function and protein synthesis, with a net reduction in somatic tissue mass.[1] Therefore, upper arm anthropometric data can indicate the status of an individual's energy and protein reserves.

The triceps skinfold measurement has been correlated with other estimates of body fat derived from radiographic, densitometric, isotope-dilution, and K^{40} counting methods, and is a relatively good indicator of the amount of body fat.[2-8] Similarly, the arm muscle circumference has been correlated with other measures of total muscle mass.[2,9,10] The upper arm circumference is, of course, a composite measure reflecting both fat and muscle mass. Because both the triceps skinfold measurement and estimate of muscle circumference may underestimate the magnitude of tissue changes in the upper arm, the use of upper arm muscle and fat area calculations have also been recommended.[11] In fact, studies in children and adults indicate that fat area measurements are systematically better indicators of fat weight than is the skinfold thickness.[12]

Additionally, upper arm anthropometry lacks sufficient sensitivity to reveal subtle, short-term changes in tissue composition. However, serial anthropometric evaluation can document comparative changes in subcutaneous fat stores and somatic protein stores during nutritional depletion and repletion.[13] Serial measurements are obviously most useful when made on long-term, stressed patients with a poor exogenous nutritional intake.

Although several surveys have documented that a significant proportion of hospitalized patients have depressed anthropometric measurements, a correlation of such measurements with morbidity and mortality in general medical or surgical patients has not been reported.[14-17] The arm muscle circumference has been reported as a significant predictor of morbidity in patients undergoing elective lower extremity orthopedic surgery.[18] This is not surprising since the reduction or prevention of skeletal muscle catabolism is of critical importance during the initiation of muscular rehabilitation in these immobilized patients.

CALCULATIONS

The arm muscle circumference and upper arm muscle and fat areas can be obtained by interpolation from published nomograms,[19] or can be calculated from triceps skinfold and arm circumference measurements as follows [2,11,20]:

Arm muscle circumference (mm) = AC − π TSF

$$\text{Upper arm muscle area (mm)}^2 = \frac{(AC - \pi\, TSF)^2}{4\,\pi}$$

$$\text{Upper arm fat area (mm)}^2 = \frac{\pi}{4} \times \left(\frac{AC}{\pi}\right)^2 - \frac{(AC - \pi\, TSF)^2}{4\pi}$$

where AC = upper arm circumference (cm); TSF = triceps skinfold (cm); and π = 3.14

STANDARDS

The utility and validity of anthropometric evaluation depends upon the use of appropriate standards for data interpretation. As already noted, standards derived from measurements taken during the United States Health and Nutritional Examination Survey of 1971 to 1974 are currently accepted as the most representative for the United States population.[11,21] Age and sex specific percentiles derived from the survey data were reported for arm circumference and triceps skinfold measurements (Tables 3 and 4) based on measurements of a cross-sectional sample of 19,097 white subjects aged 1 to 74 years.[11] Thereafter, age and sex specific percentiles were determined for arm muscle circumference, arm muscle area, and arm fat area (Tables 5 to 8). The sample was selected from a national probability sample that represented the noninstitutionalized white civilian population. The sample size for blacks was too small to be included as part of these norms. Therefore, the data given do not account for possible variation due to race or ethnic

TABLE 3. STANDARDS FOR TRICEPS SKINFOLD*

Triceps Skinfold Percentiles (mm²)

Age Group	Males							Females						
	5	10	25	50	75	90	95	5	10	25	50	75	90	95
1- 1.9	6	7	8	10	12	14	16	6	7	8	10	12	14	16
2- 2.9	6	7	8	10	12	14	15	6	8	9	10	12	15	16
3- 3.9	6	7	8	10	11	14	15	7	8	9	11	12	14	15
4- 4.9	6	6	8	9	11	12	14	7	8	8	10	12	14	16
5- 5.9	6	6	8	9	11	14	15	6	7	8	10	12	15	18
6- 6.9	5	6	7	8	10	13	16	6	6	8	10	12	14	16
7- 7.9	5	6	7	9	12	15	17	6	7	9	11	13	16	18
8- 8.9	5	6	7	8	10	13	16	6	8	9	12	15	18	24
9- 9.9	6	6	7	10	13	17	18	8	8	10	13	16	20	22
10-10.9	6	6	8	10	14	18	21	7	8	10	12	17	23	27
11-11.9	6	6	8	11	16	20	24	7	8	10	13	18	24	28
12-12.9	6	6	8	11	14	22	28	8	9	11	14	18	23	27
13-13.9	5	5	7	10	14	22	26	8	8	12	15	21	26	30
14-14.9	4	5	7	9	14	21	24	9	10	13	16	21	26	28
15-15.9	4	5	6	8	11	18	24	8	10	12	17	21	25	32
16-16.9	4	5	6	8	12	16	22	10	12	15	18	22	26	31
17-17.9	5	5	6	8	12	16	19	10	12	13	19	24	30	37
18-18.9	4	5	6	9	13	20	24	10	12	15	18	22	26	30
19-24.9	4	5	7	10	15	20	22	10	11	14	18	24	30	34
25-34.9	5	6	8	12	16	20	24	10	12	16	21	27	34	37
35-44.9	5	6	8	12	16	20	23	12	13 14	18	23	29	35	38
45-54.9	6	6	8	12	15	20	25	12	16	20	25	30	36	40
55-64.9	5	6	8	11	14	19	22	12	16	20	25	31	36	38
65-74.9	4	6	8	11	15	19	22	12	14	18	24	29	34	36

*These percentiles were derived from data obtained on all white subjects in the United States Health and Nutrition Examination Survey I, 1971–1974. (From Frisancho, A.R.: New norms of upper limb fat and muscle areas for assessment of nutrition status. Am. J. Clin. Nutr. 34: 2540, 1981.)

background. Several racial contrast studies have emphasized the leanness and distinctive lack of subcutaneous fat over the triceps area in black children and adults, and the use of these norms may therefore overestimate subcutaneous fat depletion in black individuals.[22-24] Race, age, and sex specific percentiles for blacks aged 6 to 50 years have also been published for triceps skinfold measurements from the Health and Nutritional Examination Survey. These percentiles are based on measurements done on 978 black males and 1682 black females[25] (Table 8).

Standards derived from the Health and Nutritional Examination Survey are accepted as superior to those published by the World Health Organization[15] since the latter were derived from measurements in other countries and probably underestimate average measurements for Americans. Age and sex specific percentiles have also been published from the Ten State Nutrition Survey. However, these data are not representative of the United States population, since the target population of the survey was located in geographical regions containing the highest percentage of families living in poverty. Specifically, since the

STANDARDS FOR FEMALE ARM CIRCUMFERENCE*

Age Group	Arm Circumference (mm)						
	5	10	25	50	75	90	95
1- 1.9	138	142	148	156	164	172	177
2- 2.9	142	145	152	160	167	176	184
3- 3.9	143	150	158	167	175	183	189
4- 4.9	149	154	160	169	177	184	191
5- 5.9	153	157	165	175	185	203	211
6- 6.9	156	162	170	176	187	204	211
7- 7.9	164	167	174	183	199	216	231
8- 8.9	168	172	183	195	214	247	261
9- 9.9	178	182	194	211	224	251	260
10-10.9	174	182	193	210	228	251	265
11-11.9	185	194	208	224	248	276	303
12-12.9	194	203	216	237	256	282	294
13-13.9	202	211	223	243	271	301	338
14-14.9	214	223	237	252	272	304	322
15-15.9	208	221	239	254	279	300	322
16-16.9	218	224	241	258	283	318	334
17-17.9	220	227	241	264	295	324	350
18-18.9	222	227	241	258	281	312	325
19-24.9	221	230	247	265	290	319	345
25-34.9	233	240	256	277	304	342	368
35-44.9	241	251	267	290	317	356	378
45-54.9	242	256	274	299	328	362	384
55-64.9	243	257	280	303	335	367	385
65-74.9	240	252	274	299	326	356	373

TABLE 4. STANDARDS FOR MALE ARM CIRCUMFERENCE*

Age Group	Arm Circumference (mm)						
	5	10	25	50	75	90	95
1- 1.9	142	146	150	159	170	176	183
2- 2.9	141	145	153	162	170	178	185
3- 3.9	150	153	160	167	175	184	190
4- 4.9	149	154	162	171	180	186	192
5- 5.9	153	160	167	175	185	195	204
6- 6.9	155	159	167	179	188	209	228
7- 7.9	162	167	177	187	201	223	230
8- 8.9	162	170	177	190	202	220	245
9- 9.9	175	178	187	200	217	249	257
10-10.9	181	184	196	210	231	262	274
11-11.9	186	190	202	223	244	261	280
12-12.9	193	200	214	232	254	282	303
13-13.9	194	211	228	247	263	286	301
14-14.9	220	226	237	253	283	303	322
15-15.9	222	229	244	264	284	311	320
16-16.9	244	248	262	278	303	324	343
17-17.9	246	253	267	285	308	336	347
18-18.9	245	260	276	297	321	353	379
19-24.9	262	272	288	308	331	355	372
25-34.9	271	282	300	319	342	362	375
35-44.9	278	287	305	326	345	363	374
45-54.9	267	281	301	322	342	362	376
55-64.9	258	273	296	317	336	355	369
65-74.9	248	263	285	307	325	344	355

*These percentiles were derived from data obtained on all white subjects in the United States Health and Nutrition Examination Survey I, 1971–1974. (From Frisancho, A.R.: New norms of upper limb fat and muscle areas for assessment of nutrition status. Am. J. Clin. Nutr. 34: 2542, 1981.)

TABLE 5. STANDARDS FOR MALE ARM MUSCLE CIRCUMFERENCE*

Age Group	Arm Muscle Circumference (mm)						
	5	10	25	50	75	90	95
1- 1.9	110	113	119	127	135	144	147
2- 2.9	111	114	122	130	140	146	150
3- 3.9	117	123	131	137	143	148	153
4- 4.9	123	126	133	141	148	156	159
5- 5.9	128	133	140	147	154	162	169
6- 6.9	131	135	142	151	161	170	177
7- 7.9	137	139	151	160	168	177	190
8- 8.9	140	145	154	162	170	182	187
9- 9.9	151	154	161	170	183	196	202
10-10.9	156	160	166	180	191	209	221
11-11.9	159	165	173	183	195	205	230
12-12.9	167	171	182	195	210	223	241
13-13.9	172	179	196	211	226	238	245
14-14.9	189	199	212	223	240	260	264
15-15.9	199	204	218	237	254	266	272
16-16.9	213	225	234	249	269	287	296
17-17.9	224	231	245	258	273	294	312
18-18.9	226	237	252	264	283	298	324
19-24.9	238	245	257	273	289	309	321
25-34.9	243	250	264	279	298	314	326
35-44.9	247	255	269	286	302	318	327
45-54.9	239	249	265	281	300	315	326
55-64.9	236	245	260	278	295	310	320
65-74.9	223	235	251	268	284	298	306

STANDARDS FOR FEMALE ARM MUSCLE CIRCUMFERENCE*

Age Group	Arm Muscle Circumference (mm)						
	5	10	25	50	75	90	95
1- 1.9	105	111	117	124	132	139	143
2- 2.9	111	114	119	126	133	142	147
3- 3.9	113	119	124	132	140	146	152
4- 4.9	115	121	128	136	144	152	157
5- 5.9	125	128	134	142	151	159	165
6- 6.9	130	133	138	145	154	166	171
7- 7.9	129	135	142	151	160	171	176
8- 8.9	138	140	151	160	171	183	194
9- 9.9	147	150	158	167	180	194	198
10-10.9	148	150	159	170	180	190	197
11-11.9	150	158	171	181	196	217	223
12-12.9	162	166	180	191	201	214	220
13-13.9	169	175	183	198	211	226	240
14-14.9	174	179	190	201	216	232	247
15-15.9	175	178	189	202	215	228	244
16-16.9	170	180	190	202	216	234	249
17-17.9	175	183	194	205	221	239	257
18-18.9	174	179	191	202	215	237	245
19-24.9	179	185	195	207	221	236	249
25-34.9	183	188	199	212	228	246	264
35-44.9	186	192	205	218	236	257	272
45-54.9	187	193	206	220	238	260	274
55-64.9	187	196	209	225	244	266	280
65-74.9	185	195	208	225	244	264	279

*These percentiles were derived from data obtained on all white subjects in the United States Health and Nutrition Examination Survey I, 1971–1974. (From Frisancho, A.R.: New norms of upper limb fat and muscle areas for assessment of nutrition status. Am. J. Clin. Nutr. 34: 2542, 1981.)

159

TABLE 6. STANDARDS FOR MALE UPPER ARM MUSCLE AREA*

Age Group	Arm Muscle Area Percentiles (mm²)						
	5	10	25	50	75	90	95
1- 1.9	956	1014	1133	1278	1447	1644	1720
2- 2.9	973	1040	1190	1345	1557	1690	1787
3- 3.9	1095	1201	1357	1484	1618	1750	1853
4- 4.9	1207	1264	1408	1579	1747	1926	2008
5- 5.9	1298	1411	1550	1720	1884	2089	2285
6- 6.9	1360	1447	1605	1815	2056	2297	2493
7- 7.9	1497	1548	1808	2027	2246	2494	2886
8- 8.9	1550	1664	1895	2089	2296	2628	2788
9- 9.9	1811	1884	2067	2288	2657	3053	3257
10-10.9	1930	2027	2182	2575	2903	3486	3882
11-11.9	2016	2156	2382	2670	3022	3359	4226
12-12.9	2216	2339	2649	3022	3496	3968	4640
13-13.9	2363	2546	3044	3553	4081	4502	4794
14-14.9	2830	3147	3586	3963	4575	5368	5530
15-15.9	3138	3317	3788	4481	5134	5631	5900
16-16.9	3625	4044	4352	4951	5753	6576	6980
17-17.9	3998	4252	4777	5286	5950	6886	7726
18-18.9	4070	4481	5066	5552	6374	7067	8355
19-24.9	4508	4777	5274	5913	6660	7606	8200
25-34.9	4694	4963	5541	6214	7067	7847	8436
35-44.9	4844	5181	5740	6490	7265	8034	8488
45-54.9	4546	4946	5589	6297	7142	7918	8458
55-64.9	4422	4783	5381	6144	6919	7670	8149
65-74.9	3973	4411	5031	5716	6432	7074	7453

*These percentiles were derved from data obtained on all white subjects in the United States Health and Nutrition Examination Survey I, 1971–1974. (From Frisancho, A.R.: New norms of upper limb fat and muscle areas for assessment of nutrition status. Am. J. Clin. Nutr. 34: 2543, 1981.)

STANDARDS FOR FEMALE UPPER ARM MUSCLE AREA*

Age Group	Arm Muscle Area Percentiles (mm²)						
	5	10	25	50	75	90	95
1- 1.9	885	973	1084	1221	1378	1535	1621
2- 2.9	973	1029	1119	1269	1405	1595	1727
3- 3.9	1014	1133	1227	1396	1563	1690	1846
4- 4.9	1058	1171	1313	1475	1644	1832	1958
5- 5.9	1238	1301	1423	1598	1825	2012	2159
6- 6.9	1354	1414	1513	1683	1877	2182	2323
7- 7.9	1330	1441	1602	1815	2045	2332	2469
8- 8.9	1513	1566	1808	2034	2327	2657	2996
9- 9.9	1723	1788	1976	2227	2571	2987	3112
10-10.9	1740	1784	2019	2296	2583	2873	3093
11-11.9	1784	1987	2316	2612	3071	3739	3953
12-12.9	2092	2182	2579	2904	3225	3655	3847
13-13.9	2269	2426	2657	3130	3529	4081	4568
14-14.9	2418	2562	2874	3220	3704	4294	4850
15-15.9	2426	2518	2847	3248	3689	4123	4756
16-16.9	2308	2567	2865	3248	3718	4353	4946
17-17.9	2442	2674	2996	3336	3883	4552	5251
18-18.9	2398	2538	2917	3243	3694	4461	4767
19-24.9	2538	2728	3026	3406	3877	4439	4940
25-34.9	2661	2826	3148	3573	4138	4806	5541
35-44.9	2750	2948	3359	3783	4428	5240	5877
45-54.9	2784	2956	3378	3858	4520	5375	5964
55-64.9	2784	3063	3477	4045	4750	5632	6247
65-74.9	2737	3018	3444	4019	4739	5566	6214

TABLE 7. STANDARDS FOR MALE UPPER ARM FAT AREA*

Age Group	Arm Fat Area Percentiles (mm²)						
	5	10	25	50	75	90	95
1- 1.9	452	486	590	741	895	1036	1176
2- 2.9	434	504	578	737	871	1044	1148
3- 3.9	464	519	590	736	868	1071	1151
4- 4.9	428	494	598	722	859	989	1085
5- 5.9	446	488	582	713	914	1176	1299
6- 6.9	371	446	539	678	896	1115	1519
7- 7.9	423	473	574	758	1011	1393	1511
8- 8.9	410	460	588	725	1003	1248	1558
9- 9.9	485	527	635	859	1252	1864	2081
10-10.9	523	543	738	982	1376	1906	2609
11-11.9	536	595	754	1148	1710	2348	2574
12-12.9	554	650	874	1172	1558	2536	3580
13-13.9	475	570	812	1096	1702	2744	3322
14-14.9	453	563	786	1082	1608	2746	3508
15-15.9	521	595	690	931	1423	2434	3100
16-16.9	542	593	844	1078	1746	2280	3041
17-17.9	598	698	827	1096	1636	2407	2888
18-18.9	560	665	860	1264	1947	3302	3928
19-24.9	594	743	963	1406	2231	3098	3652
25-34.9	675	831	1174	1752	2459	3246	3786
35-44.9	703	851	1310	1792	2463	3098	3624
45-54.9	749	922	1254	1741	2359	3245	3928
55-64.9	658	839	1166	1645	2236	2976	3466
65-74.9	573	753	1122	1621	2199	2876	3327

STANDARDS FOR FEMALE UPPER ARM FAT AREA*

Age Group	Arm Fat Area Percentiles (mm²)						
	5	10	25	50	75	90	95
1- 1.9	401	466	578	706	847	1022	1140
2- 2.9	469	526	642	747	894	1061	1173
3- 3.9	473	529	656	822	967	1106	1158
4- 4.9	490	541	654	766	907	1109	1236
5- 5.9	470	529	647	812	991	1330	1536
6- 6.9	464	508	638	827	1009	1263	1436
7- 7.9	491	560	706	920	1135	1407	1644
8- 8.9	527	634	769	1042	1383	1872	2482
9- 9.9	642	690	933	1219	1584	2171	2524
10-10.9	616	702	842	1141	1608	2500	3005
11-11.9	707	802	1015	1301	1942	2730	3690
12-12.9	782	854	1090	1511	2056	2666	3369
13-13.9	726	838	1219	1625	2374	3272	4150
14-14.9	981	1043	1423	1818	2403	3250	3765
15-15.9	839	1126	1396	1886	2544	3093	4195
16-16.9	1126	1351	1663	2006	2598	3374	4236
17-17.9	1042	1267	1463	2104	2977	3864	5159
18-18.9	1003	1230	1616	2104	2617	3508	3733
19-24.9	1046	1198	1596	2166	2959	4050	4896
25-34.9	1173	1399	1841	2548	3512	4690	5560
35-44.9	1336	1619	2158	2898	3932	5093	5847
45-54.9	1459	1803	2447	3244	4229	5416	6140
55-64.9	1345	1879	2520	3369	4360	5276	6152
65-74.9	1363	1681	2266	3063	3943	4914	5530

*These percentiles were derived from data obtained on all white subjects in the United States Health and Nutrition Examination Survey I, 1971–1974. (From Frisancho, A.R.: New norms of upper limb fat and muscle areas for assessment of nutrition status. Am. J. Clin. Nutr. 34: 2543, 1981.)

TABLE 8. TRICEPS SKINFOLD STANDARDS FOR BLACKS*

Triceps Skinfold Percentiles (mm)

	Male							Female						
Age	5	10	25	50	75	90	95	5	10	25	50	75	90	95
6	4.0	4.0	5.1	6.4	8.4	10.4	13.0	3.7	4.8	6.1	7.4	9.7	11.3	19.4
7	4.0	4.2	5.3	6.5	8.8	11.7	15.1	3.9	5.0	6.6	8.1	10.9	14.2	21.1
8	4.0	4.3	5.5	6.6	9.1	12.7	16.9	4.1	5.4	7.2	9.0	12.2	17.1	23.0
9	4.0	4.4	5.6	6.8	9.2	13.7	18.6	4.5	5.8	7.8	10.1	13.6	19.8	24.9
10	4.0	4.4	5.7	6.9	9.3	14.4	20.2	4.9	6.2	8.3	11.1	14.9	22.3	26.9
11	4.0	4.4	5.7	7.0	9.3	15.2	21.6	5.4	6.7	8.9	12.0	16.3	24.3	28.7
12	3.9	4.4	5.6	7.1	9.4	15.9	22.9	5.8	7.1	9.4	12.9	17.6	25.9	30.3
13	3.9	4.3	5.5	7.1	9.5	16.5	24.0	6.3	7.4	9.9	13.7	18.8	27.2	31.7
14	3.8	4.2	5.3	7.2	9.7	17.2	24.9	6.6	7.7	10.4	14.4	19.9	28.1	32.8
15	3.7	4.1	5.2	7.2	9.9	17.8	25.4	6.9	7.8	10.8	14.9	20.8	28.8	33.6
16	3.6	4.0	5.0	7.1	10.1	18.2	25.6	7.0	7.9	11.1	15.4	21.6	29.4	34.1
17	3.5	3.9	4.9	7.1	10.3	18.6	25.4	7.1	7.9	11.4	15.8	22.3	29.9	34.5
18–20	3.3	3.7	4.8	6.9	10.7	18.7	23.1	7.2	8.4	12.2	16.9	23.8	31.5	34.7
21–23	3.3	3.7	4.8	6.9	10.9	18.2	21.7	7.5	9.1	12.7	17.7	24.6	32.5	34.8
24–26	3.3	3.7	5.1	7.9	11.8	17.9	23.7	8.4	10.6	13.8	19.8	26.8	33.5	36.5
27–29	3.4	3.8	5.5	8.7	12.9	18.4	25.9	8.7	10.6	14.5	21.0	28.5	34.0	38.1
30–32	3.6	4.2	6.5	10.3	14.9	19.2	26.3	8.6	9.9	16.3	23.8	31.9	36.5	41.9
33–35	3.7	4.5	6.9	10.6	15.0	19.3	24.5	8.7	10.2	17.3	25.0	33.1	38.1	43.4
36–38	4.1	4.8	7.0	10.0	13.8	20.1	23.5	9.6	12.3	18.9	26.1	33.3	39.8	44.7
39–41	4.2	4.7	6.7	9.4	13.3	20.9	25.4	9.7	13.2	19.2	26.0	32.8	39.9	44.6
42–44	3.8	4.2	6.1	8.8	13.5	21.3	27.8	8.6	12.3	18.9	25.8	32.0	40.2	43.6
45–47	3.5	4.0	6.0	9.0	13.8	20.3	26.8	8.0	11.3	18.5	26.0	32.5	40.7	43.4
48–50	3.1	4.1	6.0	9.8	14.0	18.5	24.8	8.8	11.1	18.4	26.8	34.8	41.4	44.7

*These smoothed percentiles were derived from data obtained on black subjects in the Health and Nutrition Examination Survey I, 1971-1974. (From Cronk, C.E. and Roche, A.F.: Race and sex specific reference data for triceps and subscapular skinfolds and weight/statute. Am. J. Clin. Nutr. 35: 347, 1982.)

50th percentiles for triceps skinfold and arm circumference are generally lower in this survey than in the Health and Nutrition Examination Survey, evaluation of upper arm anthropometric measurements on hospitalized patients using these reference standards may overestimate the incidence and degree of nutritional depletion among such patients.

DATA INTERPRETATION

Upper arm measurements and calculations within the 5th to 25th percentile of standards reported from the United States Health and Nutritional Examination Survey may be considered indicative of moderate nutritional depletion, while those below the 5th percentile indicate severe nutritional depletion.[26,27] Such measurements and calculations are also commonly expressed as a percentage of a standard (the 50th percentile), and are interpreted as reflecting moderate depletion when between 60–90 percent of standard, and as reflecting severe depletion when less than 60 percent of standard.[28] However, the use of percentages fails to account for differences in variability between measurements and calculations, and the use of percentiles for data classification is therefore recommended.[29] Computerized axial tomography indicates that fat is distributed asymmetrically around the arm, and that no fat is radiologically detectable when the triceps skinfold is less than 5 mm.[30] Such a reading may therefore indicate severe and critical depletion in stressed patients.

Because fat is a dispensable tissue and the depletion of fat stores does not necessarily correlate with loss of function, protein-calorie malnutrition cannot be diagnosed solely by triceps skinfold measurements. However, a low triceps skinfold measurement does indicate depletion of the primary caloric reserve of the body, which may be critical to survival in those patients with increased energy/nutrient requirements and a simultaneously low energy/nutrient intake (i.e., with surgery, infection, sepsis, burns). In these instances the triceps skinfold measurement may indicate the need for immediate and aggressive nutritional intervention. The correlation between upper arm anthropometric measurements and total body fat and muscle contents suggests that these measurements may be useful for nutritional screening as well as for documentation of comparative changes in body stores during nutritional repletion when measured at consistent intervals. Upper arm anthropometry may be of little value for evaluating obese patients (> 150 percent of the desirable weight). Substantial variability has been reported in this index in such cases, since delineation of the skinfold is technically more difficult than in lean individuals.[31] In obese subjects, anthropometric estimates of the upper arm muscle and fat areas have been reported to differ from radiographic values by more than 50 percent.[30] Midarm computerized axial tomographic scanning provides an accurate alternative to anthropometric methods for estimating midarm muscle and fat in obese individuals.

The practitioner should also be cognizant of the limitations inherent in upper arm anthropometry when interpreting the data. Calculations of upper arm fat and muscle areas are only approximations, since the formulas utilized are based on the idealized assumptions (the upper arm is cylindrical in form and has an even distribution of fat) which are subject to some inaccuracy. Additionally, the estimate of fat area does not adjust for variable skinfold compressibility. Changes in skin compressibility with age have been reported.[32] Furthermore, estimates of muscle mass do not take into account the humeral diameter, any variation in which is therefore not included.[11] In particular, since bone area is not influenced appreciably by nutritional status, calculations of arm muscle area may underestimate the degree of muscle atrophy in malnutrition.[30] However, a radiographic study of the arm composition of white children reported the same ratio of muscle to bone in both sexes before and after adolescence, suggesting that bone and muscle increase proportionately during growth.[33]

Although the foregoing considerations are of little concern in evaluations of anthropometric data for nutritional screening purposes or to detect serial changes in nutritional status, recognition of the limitations of indirect derivation is warranted when classifying the degree of nutritional depletion and planning subsequent therapy in a particular case.

REFERENCES

1. Wilmore, D.: The Metabolic Management of the Critically Ill. Plenum Book Co., New York, 1977.
2. Jelliffe, D.B.: The Assessment of Nutritional Status of the Community. W.H.O. Monograph No. 53, 1966.
3. Foman, S.J.: Nutritional Disorders of Children: Prevention, Screening and Follow-up. DHEW Publication No. (HSA) 78-5104, 1978.
4. Brozek, J.: Physique and nutritional status of adult men. Hum. Biol. 28:124, 1956.
5. Tanner, J.M.: The measurement of body fat in man. Proc. Nutr. Soc. 18:148, 1959.
6. Ward, G.M., Krzywicki, H.J., Rahman, D.P., Quaas, R.L., Nelson, R.A. and Consolazio, C.F.: Relationship of anthropometric measurements to body fat as determined by densitometry, potassium–40, and body water. Am. J. Clin. Nutr. 28:162, 1975.
7. Mayer, J.: Obesity. In Modern Nutrition in Health and Disease, 5th ed. Goodhart, R.S. and Shils, M.E. (eds). Lea and Febiger, Philadelphia, 1973.
8. Cahill, G.F.: Starvation in man. N. Engl. J. Med. 282:668, 1970.
9. Standard, K.L., Wills, V.G., and Waterlow, J.C.: Indirect indicators of muscle mass in malnourished infants. Am. J. Clin. Nutr. 7:271, 1959.
10. Reindorp, S. and Whitehead, R.G.: Changes in serum creatinine kinase and other biological measurements associated with musculature in children recovering from Kwashiorkor. Br. J. Nutr. 25:273, 1971.
11. Frisancho, A.R.: New norms of upper limb fat and muscle areas for assessment of nutritional status. Am. J. Clin. Nutr. 34:2540, 1981.
12. Hines, J.H., Roche, A.F., and Webb, P.: Fat areas as estimates of total body fat. Am. J. Clin. Nutr. 33:2093, 1980.
13. Faintuch, J., Faintuch, J.J., Machade, M.C., et al.: Anthropometric assessment of nutritional depletion after surgical injury. JPEN 5:359, 1979.
14. Bistrian, B.R., Blackburn, G.L., Hallowell, E., et al.: Protein status of general surgical patients. JAMA 230:858–860, 1974.
15. Bistrian, B.R., Blackburn, G.L., Vitale, J., et al.: Prevalence of malnutrition in general medical patients. JAMA 235:1567, 1976.
16. Hill, G.L., Blacket, R.L., Rickford, I., et al.: Malnutrition in surgical patients: An unrecognized problem. Lancet 1:689, 1977.
17. Kassiadou, A., Domingos, J.C., Ronaldo, V., et al.: Malnutrition in general medical and surgical patients: An anthropometric survey in Niteroi, Brazil, JPEN 3:470, 1979.
18. Jensen, J.E., Jensen, T.G., Smith, T.K., et al.: Nutrition in orthopaedic surgery. J. Bone and Joint Surg. 64A:1263, 1983.
19. Gurney, J.M. and Jelliffe, D.B.: Arm anthropometry in nutritional assessment: Nomogram for rapid calculation of muscle circumference and cross-sectional muscle and fat areas. Am. J. Clin. Nutr. 26:912, 1973.
20. Frisancho, A.R.: Triceps skinfold and upper arm muscle size: Norms for evaluation of nutritional status. Am. J. Clin. Nutr. 27:1052, 1974.
21. Bishop, C.W., Bowen, P.E., and Ritchey, S.J.: Norms for nutritional assessment in American adults by upper arm anthropometry. Am. J. Clin. Nutr. 34:25, 1981.
22. Robson, J.P., Bazin, M., and Soderstrom, R.: Ethnic differences in skinfold thickness. Am. J. Clin. Nutr. 24:864, 1971.
23. Malina, R.M.: Skinfolds in American negro and white children. J. Am. Diet. Assoc. 53:34, 1971.
24. Malina, R.M.: Skinfold–body weight correlations in negro and white children of elementary school age. Am. J. Clin. Nutr. 25:861, 1972.
25. Cronk, C.E. and Roche, A.F.: Race and sex-specific reference data for triceps and subscapular skinfolds and weight/stature. Am. J. Clin. Nutr. 35:347, 1982.

26. Gray, G.E. and Gray, L.K.: Validity of anthropometric norms used in the assessment of hospitalized patients. JPEN 3:366, 1979.

27. Gray, G.E. and Gray, L.K.: Anthropometric measurements and their interpretation: principles, practices, problems. J. Am. Diet. Assoc. 77:534, 1980.

28. Blackburn, G.L., Bistrian, B.R., Mani, B.S., et al.: Nutritional and metabolic assessment of the hospitalized patient. JPEN 1:11, 1979.

29. Burgert, S.L. and Anderson, C.F.: An evaluation of upper arm measurements used in nutritional assessment. Am. J. Clin. Nutr. 32:2136, 1976.

30. Heymsfield, S.V., Olafson, R.P., Kutner, M.H., et al.: A radiographic method of quantifying protein-calorie undernutrition. Am. J. Clin. Nutr. 32:693, 1979.

31. Bray, G.A., Greenway, F.L., Molich, M.E., et al.: Use of anthropometric measures to assess weight loss. Am. J. Clin. Nutr. 31:769, 1978.

32. Clegg, E.F. and Kent, C.: Skinfold compressibility of young adults. Hum. Biol. 39: 1977.

33. Malina, R.M. and Johnson, F.E.: Relations between bone, muscle and fat widths in the upper arms and calves of boys and girls studied cross-sectionally at ages 6–16 years. Hum. Biol. 39:211, 1967.

C. Creatinine/Height Index

In severe cases of protein malnutrition, tissue analyses indicate that liver and muscle may lose up to 50 percent of their cytoplasmic mass.[1] Because muscle is the largest protein-containing tissue in the body, indices of the somatic muscle mass provide useful data for evaluating the degree of protein depletion.

Active muscle elaborates free creatinine at a relatively constant rate in proportion to the muscle mass under circumstances of normal renal function and sufficient fluid intake.[2] Free creatinine is an anhydride of muscle creatine formed by an irreversible reaction, and is solely a waste product of creatine; thus, approximately 2 percent of muscle creatine is transformed into creatinine every 24 hours.[3] In normal adults, any increase in the serum creatinine level that might occur from an increase in body size should be offset by an increase in creatinine excretion, thus rendering the serum level constant. With chronic wasting disease, both the skeletal muscle mass and creatinine excretion decrease simultaneously.[4-8]

A significant correlation between the 24-hour creatinine excretion, basal oxygen consumption, and lean body mass as measured by specific gravity has been demonstrated in a group of adults.[9] The rate of endogenous creatinine production is directly related to the amount of lean muscle mass, so that a positive linear correlation exists between the daily urinary creatinine excretion and the body weight, body surface area, and height.[10] Urinary creatinine excretion has also been significantly correlated with arm and thigh muscle circumference and with x-ray muscle shadow weights.[4,5] Finally, several investigators have reported that children with protein-calorie malnutrition have a significantly reduced urinary creatinine excretion which increases with adequate nutritional therapy.[4,11] A significant correlation between the total body potassium content and creatinine excretion, based on K^{40} measurements, has been reported.[12,13] These findings indicate that creatinine excretion reflects the total lean body mass in malnourished individuals as well as normal children and adults.

Since height remains essentially unchanged by malnutrition, while creatinine excretion continues to correlate with body cell mass, the creatinine/height index affords a means of assessing the nutritional status of metabolically active tissue by allowing the expected body cell mass-for-height to be compared with the actual body cell mass. However, since the arm muscle circumference correlates closely with creatinine excretion, the creatinine/height index is usually employed for the comprehensive and serial evaluation of malnourished patients rather than as a routine screening procedure.

Although serial tests will detect further depletion, positive responses to nutritional therapy during short-term hospitalization may not be detected since some physical activity is essential to the synthesis of lean body mass.[14,15]

To date, depressed creatinine/height index calculations have not been significantly correlated with increased morbidity or mortality in hospitalized patients.

METHODOLOGY AND CALCULATION

Determination of the urinary creatinine excretion requires the collection of a 24-hour urine specimen for analysis (Section II-M). However, the need for timed 24-hour—and preferably 72-hour—urine collection for the determination limits its practicality; methods which involve the collection of a 3-hour sample have been reported as alternatives. However, the coefficient of variation of the creatinine/height index increases inversely as the collection time decreases[16] (Table 9), and three consecutive 24-hour specimens are recommended to reduce variation. A coefficient of variation of 7 percent is considered highly satisfactory, since the urinary creatinine determination itself has a coefficient of variation of 2.6 percent.[7]

The creatinine/height index (in percent) is calculated as follows:

$$\text{CHI} \% = \frac{\text{mg creatinine excreted by patient}/24\,\text{hours}}{\text{mg creatinine excreted by normal subject of same height}/24\,\text{hours}} \times 100.$$

TABLE 9. COEFFICIENT OF VARIATION OF THE CREATININE/HEIGHT INDEX FOR VARIOUS TIMED URINE COLLECTIONS

Duration of Urine Collection Period	Coefficient of Variation of Creatinine/Height Index
3 hour	25.6%
8 hour	18.5%
24 hour	13.3%
48 hour	9.0%
72 hour	6.9%

(From Viteri, F.E., Alvarado, J. and Alleyne, G.A.O.: Am. J. Clin. Nutr. 24: 386, 1971.)

TABLE 10. IDEAL URINARY CREATININE VALUES

Men*		Women**	
Height (cm)	Ideal Creatinine (mg)	Height (cm)	Ideal Creatinine (mg)
157.5	1288	147.3	830
160.0	1325	149.9	851
162.6	1359	152.4	875
165.1	1386	154.9	900
167.6	1426	157.5	925
170.2	1467	160.0	949
172.7	1513	162.6	977
175.3	1555	165.1	1006
177.8	1596	167.6	1044
180.3	1642	170.2	1076
182.9	1691	172.7	1109
185.4	1739	175.3	1141
188.0	1785	177.8	1174
190.5	1831	180.3	1206
193.0	1891	182.9	1240

*Creatinine coefficient (men) = 23 mg/kg of ideal body weight.
**Creatinine coefficient (women) = 18 mg/kg of ideal body weight.
(From Blackburn, G.L. et al: Nutritional and metabolic assessment of the hospitalized patient. J P E N 1:11–21, 1977.)

STANDARDS

Tables of expected 24-hour urinary creatinine excretions for men and women have been published.[8,17,18] These tables list the expected daily creatinine excretion by a small number of subjects for a given height and sex (Table 10). The creatinine-excretion standards that have been established are products of the average creatinine excretion rate and the ideal body weight for a given height and sex. In men, the ideal creatinine excretion has been reported as 23 mg per kilogram of the ideal body weight for a given height per 24 hours. The ideal creatinine excretion for women is 18 mg per kilogram of the ideal body weight for a given height per 24 hours.[17] There is obviously a need for larger surveys which will provide data for subjects from all age groups.

DATA INTERPRETATION

Lean body mass is depleted during malnutrition as muscle protein is catabolized for energy production and maintenance of visceral proteins, and both creatinine excretion and the creatinine/height index are lowered as a result. The range of 90 to 100 percent of the standard creatinine/height index is generally accepted as normal.[8] A creatinine/height index of less than 40 percent of the standard indicates severe nutritional depletion, while an index of 40 to 90 percent of the standard is interpreted as moderate depletion.[8]

Creatinine/height index determinations are invalid in patients with an impaired urine output, since the test assumes normal renal function and urine output. Obviously, amputation renders the standard creatinine/height index useless. Additionally, the practitioner, when interpreting data, should be aware that the creatinine pool can change independently of lean body mass. Moreover, although creatinine excretion is usually considered to be relatively constant in a given individual, severe exercise and a high meat diet will cause significantly increased creatinine excretion,[3,19] and age and fever have also been reported to influence creatinine excretion.[20,21] A decline in renal function and creatinine production with aging has been described.[22-26] Renal glomular filtration decreases, resulting in a gradually decreasing creatinine clearance;[25,26] this may be offset by a decrease in creatinine production due to the age-related loss of muscle mass. Therefore, the 24-hour urinary excretion of creatinine will be reduced in the elderly. A decline from 23.6 mg/kg/24 hours in 18- to 29-year-old subjects to 12.1 mg/kg/24 hours in 80-to 92-year-old subjects has been documented.[24] Therefore, if standards developed for young adults are used to calculate the creatinine/height index, the severity of somatic protein depletion for the geriatric age group may be highly overestimated.

The use of steroids will elevate creatinine excretion, reducing its value as an index of lean body mass, and a number of other medications, such as Tobramycin Sulfate and Mandol, also decrease creatinine clearance. Still other medications, such as methadone, interfere with urination by exerting an antidiuretic effect. Therefore, a medication history must be taken into consideration when interpreting creatinine/height index calculations for nutritional assessment purposes.

REFERENCES

1. Waterlow, J.C.: The protein content of liver and muscle as a measure of protein deficiency in human subjects. West Indian Med. J. 5:167, 1956.
2. Kaminski, M.V. and Jeejeebboy, K.: Unit 1 Nutritional assessment— Diagnosis of malnutrition and selection of therapy. J. Surg. Practice. May/June: 49, 1979.
3. Woo, J., Treuting, J.J., and Cannon, D.C.: Metabolic intermediates and inorganic ions. In: Clinical Diagnosis and Management, 16th Ed. Henry, J.D. (ed). W.B. Saunders and Co., Philadelphia, 1977.
4. Standard K.L., Wills, V.G., and Waterlow, J.C.: Indirect indicators of muscle mass in malnourished infants. Am. J. Clin. Nutr. 7:271, 1959.
5. Reindorp, S. and Whitehead, R.G.: Changes in serum creatinine kinase and other biological measurements associated with musculature in children recovering from Kwashiorkor. Br. J. Nutr. 25:273, 1973.
6. Forbes, G.B. and Bruining, G.J.: Urinary creatinine excretion and lean body mass. Am. J. Clin. Nutr. 29:1359, 1976.
7. Viteri, F.E. and Alvardo, J.: The creatinine/height index: Its use in the estimation of the degree of protein depletion and repletion in protein-calorie malnourished children. Pediatrics 46:696, 1979.
8. Blackburn, G.L., Bistrian, B.R., Mani, B.S., et al.: Nutritional and metabolic assessment of the hospitalized patient. JPEN 1:11, 1979.
9. Miller, A.T. and Blyth, C.S.: Estimation of lean body mass and body fat from basal oxygen consumption and creatinine excretion. J. Appl. Physiol. 5:73, 1952.
10. Greenblatt, D.J., Ransil, B.J., Harmatz, J.S., et al.: Variability of 24-hour urinary creatinine excretion by normal subjects. J. Clin. Pharmacol. 16:321, 1976.
11. Arroyave, G., Wilson, D., Behar, M., et al.: Serum and urinary creatinine in children with severe protein malnutrition. Am. J. Clin. Nutr. 9:176, 1961.

12. Muldowney, F.P., Crooks, J., and Bluhm, M.M.: The relationship of total exchangeable potassium and chloride to lean body mass, red cell mass and creatinine excretion in man. J. Clin. Invest. 36:1375, 1957.

13. Alleyne, G.A.O.: Studies on total body potassium in infantile malnutrition: The relationship of body fluid spaces and urinary creatinine. Clin. Sci. 34:199, 1968.

14. Deutrick, J.E., Wheldon, G.D., and Shorr, E.: Effects of immobilization upon various metabolic and physiologic functions of normal men. Am. J. Med. 4:3, 1948.

15. Umpathy, K.P., Mack, P.B., Dozier, E.A.: Effect of immobilization on urinary excretion of creatine and creatinine with certain possible ameliorating measured applied.

16. Viteri, F.E., Alvarado, J., and Alleyne, G.A.O.: Letter to the editor. Am. J. Clin. Nutr. 24:386, 1971.

17. Bistrian, B.R., Blackburn, G.L. and Shermann, M., et al.: Therapeutic index of nutritional depletion in hospitalized patients. Surg. Gynecol. Obstet. 141:512, 1975.

18. Grant, A.: Section D. Laboratory assessment of nutritional status. In Nutritional Assessment Guidelines. Cutter Medical, 1979, pp. 39–40.

19. Bleiler, R.A. and Schedl, H.P.: Creatinine excretion: Variability and relationship to diet and body size. J. Lab. Clin. Med. 59:945, 1962.

20. Pansil, B.J., Greenblatt, D.J., and Koch-Weser, J.: Evidence for systematic temporal variation in 24-hour urinary creatinine excretion. J. Clin. Pharmacol. 17:108, 1977.

21. Driver, A.J. and McAlevy, M.T.: Creatinine/height index as a function of age. Am. J. Clin. Nutr. 33:2057, 1980.

22. Doolan, P.D., Alpen, E.L., and Theil, G.B.: A clinical appraisal of the plasma concentration and endogenous clearance of creatinine. Am. J. Med. 32:65, 1962.

23. Sursback-Nielson, K., Hansen, J.M., Kampman, J., et al.: Rapid evaluation of creatinine clearance. Lancet 1:1133, 1971.

24. Crockroft, D.W. and Gault, M.H. Prediction of creatinine clearance from serum creatinine. Nephron 16:31, 1976.

25. Paper, S.: The effects of age in reducing renal function. Geriatrics 28:83, 1973.

26. Mitchell, C.O. and Lipschitz, D.A. Detection of protein-calorie malnutrition in the elderly. Am. J. Clin. Nutr. 35:398, 1982.

D. Serum Albumin

Albumin is the major hepatically synthesized transport protein of the body; it functions primarily to provide oncotic pressure and to carry long-chain fatty acids, bilirubin, calcium, metal ions, drugs, and vitamins.[1]

The serum albumin concentration is the complex net result of synthesis, degradation, and distribution of albumin. However, only 30 to 40 percent of the total exchangeable albumin pool is located in the serum compartment. The skin contains 30 to 40 percent of the total extravascular albumin, while the remainder is distributed in lower concentrations throughout the muscles and viscera. During protein deprivation, albumin levels in the serum may require days or weeks to decrease as a result of redistribution of extravascular albumin into the plasma pool.[1-3]

Nutrition is the most important factor regulating albumin synthesis since adequate nitrogen intake is basic to all other protein synthesis mechanisms. During experimental dietary protein depletion, a reduction in the rate of albumin synthesis is observed, presumably through a reduction in the availability of amino acids. Meanwhile, albumin catabolism continues at a normal rate, so that a gradual reduction in the albumin pool size and serum concentration results. After a latent period, there is a reduction in the albumin catabolic rate as the body attempts to conserve the albumin pool until synthesis returns the pool to its normal levels.[2,4]

Because of these conserving processes, as well as the large body pool and relatively long serum half-life of 20 days, the serum albumin concentration decreases slowly during malnutrition. This decrease may represent a late manifestation of protein deficiency which is often associated with clinically overt signs of malnutrition.[5] The total exchangeable albumin pool may decrease to one-third of its normal levels before the appearance of a decreased serum albumin concentration.[2] The serum albumin concentration is recognized as a valid measure of nutritional status in epidemiologic surveys.[5-7] Additionally, the serum albumin concentration has been used as a clinical screening indicator of nutritional status in hospitals, since it is readily accessible, its measurement is routinely ordered, and it correlates with increased morbidity rates.[8-10] Some evidence suggests that serum albumin levels may decrease even before anthropometric measurements indicate depletion.[11] Significant correlations between the body cell mass and serum albumin levels have been reported, supporting use of the serum albumin concentration to screen patients for nutritional problems.[6,7]

Surveys done on selected patient populations in acute- and chronic-care facilities have documented a high incidence of hypoalbuminemia before and/or during hospitalization.[12-18] Additionally, hypoalbuminemia has been correlated repeatedly with increased morbidity and mortality rates. At one teaching hospital in New Jersey,[8] statistically significant correlations were reported between depressed albumin and lymphocyte levels and patient morbidity (a fourfold increase) and mortality (a sixfold increase) in 500 consecutive adult admissions. The serum albumin concentration has also been identified as a prognostic indicator for morbidity and mortality in a surgical patient population,[9,10] and in one study, surgical intensive care unit patients with depressed albumin levels and lymphocyte counts were reported to have twice the complication rate and 4.5 times the death rate of SICU patients with normal albumin levels and lymphocyte counts.[19] Lewis and Klein identified preoperative hypoalbuminemia and a low total lymphocyte count as risk factors for postoperative sepsis in patients admitted for gastric and colonic operations.[20] Reinhardt et al. reported a linear correlation between the level of hypoalbuminemia observed in a population of 2060 hospitalized veterans and the subsequent 30-day mortality rate in this group,[21] while Bienia et al. correlated low serum albumin levels with other indicators of malnutrition with an increased rate of infection and increased mortality rate in alcoholic and nonalcoholic hospitalized veterans.[22] A serum albumin concentration of less than 3.0 g/dl was indentified as an indicator of imminent bacteremic sepsis in thermally injured patients who were evaluated on the tenth postburn day.[23]

However, lack of sensitivity and specificity limit the use of serum albumin measurements as sole or primary indicators of an individual's nutritional status.[5] Sequential albumin determinations to evaluate changes in nutritional status may also be of limited value, since significant changes in this status may be accompanied by minimal changes in the serum albumin concentration. The stability of serum albumin concentrations is explained by the large total albumin pool, the capacity of the liver to maintain albumin synthesis, and the body's ability to alter albumin distribution and reduce albumin catabolism.

METHOD

Because serum albumin is a stable protein with minimal heterogeneity, it is easily analyzed by a variety of chemical and immunologic methods and is routinely measured in hospital laboratories. The capacity of albumin to bind and transport small molecules is exploited in widely used dye-binding assay methods for this protein (such as those that use Bromcresol green (BCG), methyl orange, and 2, 4-hydroxyazobenzene-benzoic acid).[24] These techniques compare favorably with electrophoretic methods and are simpler and more easily automated. The BCG dye-binding method is recognized as superior to other dye-binding methods because of its freedom from drug interference; to date, no medically used drugs have been shown to interfere with the serum quantitation of albumin by this method. However, serum samples from highly icteric patients, and those with hemoglobin concentrations of greater than 500 mg/dl may interfere with albumin determinations done with the BCG method.[25]

STANDARDS/NORMAL RANGE

The normal mean concentration of serum albumin in adults is 4.2 g/dl, with a range of 3.5 to 5.0 g/dl.[2] However, normal ranges for albumin should be verified by each hospital laboratory in accordance with the methodology used for determinations.

DATA INTERPRETATION

A serum albumin concentration of less than 3.4 g/dl warrants further nutritional evaluation. Serum albumin concentrations below 3.0 g/dl are often associated with hypoalbuminemic edema,[5] while concentrations of less than 2.5 g/dl are extreme and indicate severe depletion, and those below 1.5 g/dl are considered critically low.

Many factors other than an inadequate nutrient intake may cause or contribute to a low serum albumin concentration. Consideration of these factors is imperative when interpreting data and planning subsequent nutritional therapy. Reductions in the body's albumin pool, which are usually reflected by changes in the serum albumin concentration, are the net result of one or a combination of three separate mechanisms: decreased synthesis, increased degradation, or excessive loss, any one of which can be caused by disease. In clinical medicine, hypoalbuminemia is generally not the result of a single mechanism.

Decreased albumin synthesis may be caused by malnutrition, liver disease, congenital analbuminemia, or hormonal factors. Albumin synthesis rates are highly dependent upon the supply of amino acids in the diet, and anorexia, inanition, and starvation undoubtedly contribute to the reduced albumin levels seen in many diseases. With fasting or the consumption of a protein-deficient diet, there is a significant slowing of albumin synthesis, even with an adequate caloric intake.[26,27] Liver disease, usually cirrhosis, is probably the most common clinical condition associated with hypoalbuminemia. In addition to intrinsic liver disease, hypoalbuminemia in cirrhotic patients may represent a combination of such other factors as the toxic effects of alcohol,[24] abnormalities in albumin distribution, hormonal changes, and malnutrition.[1] Abnormalities in albumin distribution are particularly important in cirrhotic patients with ascites, in whom as much albumin may exist in the ascitic fluid as in the plasma. Congenital analbuminemia is an extremely rare condition that is characterized by an almost complete absence of albumin from the serum as a result of a significant decrease in the rate of synthesis of this protein.[29,30]

The increased degradation of albumin is a primary mechanism that results in hypoalbuminemia in idiopathic edema[31] and such other miscellaneous disorders as familial idiopathic hypercatabolic hypoproteinemia and the Wiskott-Aldrich syndrome.[32]

Increased exogenous loss of albumin may occur through the kidney (nephrotic syndrome), the gastrointestinal tract (protein-losing enteropathies), or the skin (acute thermal burns or eczema).

In the nephrotic syndrome, abnormal capillary filtration permits a greatly increased quantity of protein to pass into the urine. The resorptive capacity of the tubules is reduced and proteinuria develops. This urinary loss of protein initiates a reduction in the size of the total exchangeable albumin pool.[33]

Increased loss of albumin through the gastrointestinal tract occurs in two main types of disorders: (1) those related to lymphatic blockage, including constrictive pericarditis, essential telangiectasia, and mesenteric lymphatic blockage due to a tumor; and (2) diseases in which there is mucosal weeping, a direct loss of serum, or malabsorption such as in protein-losing enteropathies and inflammatory bowel disease.[34] Specific conditions such as hypertrophic gastritis or gastric polyps may also be associated with a large direct loss of albumin.[1]

The changes in albumin metabolism that occur in patients with severe burns represent a complex interaction of a number of factors. Most important is the loss of albumin from the burned area as a result of increased capillary permeability. An amount of albumin equivalent to that in the plasma pool may be lost from the body and an equal amount sequestered from the intravascular space during the first four postburn days.[35] Because the lymphatics are saturated with burn debris, they are unable to return extravascular albumin to the plasma. Loss of skin in the severely burned patient also results in a decrease in the exchangeable albumin pool. In very severe burns, anorexia may result in decreased substrate, liver damage, and an altered capacity for albumin synthesis.

Hypoalbuminemia of a slight degree frequently occurs in patients with congestive heart failure, but this decrease is due to an increase in the circulating plasma volume; cardiac disease per se does not alter the synthetic capacity of the liver.[2]

Several hormones also exert specific effects on albumin synthesis.[36] Albumin synthesis is decreased by removal of the pituitary, adrenal, or thyroid glands, whereas anabolic hormones, such as testosterone, insulin, and growth hormone, increase albumin synthesis rates.[1] Corticosteroids cause a change in the distribution of albumin which results in shift of extravascular albumin into the intravascular spaces.[1] The stress of extreme catastrophic events, such as shock, results in a decreased rate of albumin synthesis which may be partially due to liver damage. Concentrations of serum albumin are depressed in zinc-deficient patients, in whom the levels have been shown to improve or be corrected with zinc supplementation.[37]

REFERENCES

1. Rothschild, M.A., Oratz, M., and Schneider, S.S.: Albumin synthesis. Part I. N. Engl. J. Med. 286:748, 1972.
2. Taville, T.S.: Progress report: The synthesis and degradation of liver produced proteins. Gut 13:225–241, 1972.
3. Rothschild, M.A., Oratz, M., and Schneider, S.S.: Albumin synthesis. II. N. Engl. J. Med. 286:816, 1972.
4. Kirsch, R., Frith, L., Black, E., et al.: Regulation of albumin synthesis and catabolism by alteration of dietary protein. Nature 217:587, 1968.
5. Whitehead, R.G., Coward, W.A., and Cunn, P.J.: Serum albumin and the onset of Kwashiorkor. Lancet 1:63, 1979.
6. Forse, R.A. and Shizgal, H.M.: Serum albumin and nutritional status. JPEN 4:450–454, 1980.
7. Coward, W.A., Whitehead, R.G., and Lunn, P.G.: Reasons why hypoalbuminemia may or may not appear in protein-energy malnutrition. Br. J. Nutr. 38:115, 1977.
8. Seltzer, M.H., Bastidas, J.A., Cooper, D.M., et al.: Instant nutritional assessment. JPEN 3:157, 1979.
9. Mullen, J.L., Gertner, M.H., Buzby, G.P., et al.: Implications of malnutrition in the surgical patient. Arch. Surg. 114:121, 1979.
10. Harvey, K.B., Ruggier, I.A., Regan, C.S., et al.: Hospital morbidity-mortality risk factors using nutritional assessment. Am. J. Clin. Nutr. 31:703, 1978.
11. Young, G.A., Chem, C., and Hill, G.L.: Assessment of protein-calorie malnutrition in surgical patients from plasma proteins and anthropometric measurements. Am. J. Clin. Nutr. 31:435, 1981.
12. Hill, G.L., Blacket, R.L., Rickford, I., et al.: Malnutrition in surgical patients—An unrecognized problem. Lancet 1:689–692, 1977.
13. Weinseir, R.L., Hunker, E.M., Krumdieck, C.L., et al.: Hospital malnutrition: A prospective evaluation of general medicine patients during the course of hospitalization. Am. J. Clin. Nutr. 32:418–426, 1979.
14. Willard, M.D.: Protein-calorie malnutrition in a community hospital. JAMA 243:1720, 1980.
15. Bistrian, B.R., Blackburn, G.L., Vitale, J. et al.: Prevalence of malnutrition in general medical patients. JAMA 235:1567, 1976.
16. Bistrian, B.R., Blackburn, G.L., Hallowell, E. et al.: Protein status of general surgical patients. JAMA 230:858–860, 1974.
17. Reinhardt, G.F., Myscofski, J.W., Wilkens, D.B., et al.: Incidence of hypoalbuminemia in a hospitalized veteran population. JPEN 4:81, 1980. (Abstr).
18. Bollot, A.J. and Owens, S.D.: Evaluation of nutritional status of selected hospitalized patients. Am. J. Clin. Nutr. 26:931–938, 1973.
19. Seltzer, M.H., Fletcher, H.S., Slocum, B.A., et al.: Instant nutritional assessment in an intensive care unit. JPEN 5:70, 1981.
20. Lewis, T.R. and Klein, H.: Risk factors in postoperative sepsis: Significance of pre-operative lymphocytopenia. J. Surg. Res. 26:365, 1979.
21. Reinhardt, G.F., Myscofski, J.W., Wilkens, D.B., et al.: Incidence of mortality of hypoalbuminemic patients in hospitalized veterans. JPEN 4:357, 1980.
22. Bienia, R., Ratcliff, S., Barbour, G.L., et al.: Malnutrition and hospital prognosis in the alcoholic patient. JPEN 6:301, 1982.
23. Morath, M.A., Miller, S.F., and Finley, R.F.: Nutritional indicators of postburn bacteremic sepsis. JPEN 5:488, 1981.
24. Ritchie, R.F. Specific proteins. In: Clinical Diagnosis and Management by Laboratory Methods, 16th Ed. Henry, J.B. (ed.). W.B. Saunders Co., Philadelphia, 1979, p. 228.
25. Grant, G.H. and Kachmar, J.F.: The proteins in body fluids. In: Fundamentals of Clinical Chemistry. Tietz N. (ed.). W.B. Saunders Co., Philadelphia, 1976, p. 335.

26. Hoffenberg, R., Black, E., and Brock, J.F.: Albumin and gamma-globulin tracer studies in protein depleted states. J. Clin. Invest. 45:143, 1966.

27. James, W.P. and Hay, A.M.: Albumin metabolism: Effects of nutritional state and dietary protein intake. J. Clin. Invest. 47:1958, 1968.

28. Rubin, E. and Liber, C.S.: Alcohol-induced hepatic injury in nonalcoholic volunteers. N. Engl. J. Med. 278:869, 1968.

29. Waldmann, T.A., Gordon, R.S., and Rosse, W.: Studies on metabolism of the serum proteins and lipids in a patient with analbuminemia. Am. J. Med. 37:960, 1964.

30. Montgomery, D.A., Neill, D.W., and Dowdle, E.G.: Idiopathic hypo-analbuminemia. Clin. Sci. 22:141, 1962.

31. Gill, J.R., Jr., Cox, J., Deka, C.S., et al.: Idiopathic edema. II. Pathogenesis of edema in patients with hypoalbuminemia. Am. J. Med. 52:452, 1972.

32. Stober, W., Blaese, R.M., and Waldman, T.A.: Abnormalities of Immunoglobulin Metabolism. In: Plasma Protein Metabolism. Rothschild, M.A. and Waldman, T.A. (eds.). Academic Press, New York, 1970, p. 287.

33. Beathard, G.A.: Proteinuria and the nephrotic syndrome. Tex. Med. 69:51, 1973.

34. Waldmann, T.A.: Protein-losing enteropathy. Gastroenterology 50:422, 1966.

35. Birke, G.: Regulation of protein metabolism in burns. In: Plasma Protein Metabolism. Rothschild, M.A. and Waldmann, T.A. (eds.). Academic Press, New York, 1970, p. 415.

36. Rothschild, M.A. and Schneider, S.S.: Serum albumin. Am. J. Digest. Dis. 14:711, 1969.

37. Bates, J. and McClain, C.J.: The effect of zinc deficiency on serum concentrations of albumin, transferrin and prealbumia in man. Am. J. Clin. Nutr. 34:1655, 1981.

E. Serum Transferrin

Transferrin (siderophilin), like albumin, is a hepatically synthesized transport glycoprotein whose major physiologic function is to bind and transport ferric iron; in this process, each molecule of transferrin binds with two molecules of iron. The 30 milligrams of iron required each day for hemoglobin synthesis can be received by transferrin either near the absorptive surfaces of the GI tract or in proximity to the sites of hemoglobin degradation in the body. Transferrin delivers iron to hemoglobin and iron-containing enzyme-synthesis sites. More than 99 percent of serum iron—about 110 mg/dl—is bound to transferrin. However, only one-third of serum transferrin is normally bound with iron. The total transferrin pool acts as a cushion to buffer large amounts of absorbed or released iron that would otherwise be toxic in the free, trivalent form. Transferrin may also play an important role in trace-element transport.[1,2]

Transferrin has also been attributed to have an important role in bacteriostasis, since trivalent iron is necessary for bacterial survival and replication. Individuals with low serum iron and high transferrin levels and a high total iron binding capacity (TIBC) have been reported to be able to fight infection despite anemia, whereas those with low serum transferrin levels have been reported more susceptible to bacterial infection, and patients with congenital atransferrinemia have died of sepsis.[2]

Because transferrin has a shorter half-life (four to eight days) than albumin, and equilibrates rapidly due to small extravascular stores, nutritional depletion may result in depressed levels of this protein before changes in the serum albumin level can occur.[3,4] Documentation of depressed serum transferrin concentrations in severe protein-calorie malnutrition is conclusive. Its usefulness in the diagnosis of subclinical malnutrition is controversial, since the serum transferrin concentration varies over a wide range even in clinically obvious cases and the response to treatment is somewhat unpredictable.[4-6]

The serum transferrin concentration has been correlated with clinical outcome in several clinical studies. Kaminski et al. recently reported that patients with admission transferrin levels of less than 170 mg/dl had a two-and-one-half-fold increase in mortality when compared with patients with normal admission transferrin levels.[7] Harvey et al. reported the serum transferrin concentration to correlate positively with an anergic response to recall skin antigen testing and with subsequent mortality in a group of patients referred for nutritional support.[8] Serum transferrin concentrations of less than 150 mg/dl have been reported to predict imminent septic episodes in thermally injured patients when measured on the tenth postburn day.[9] Bienia et al. reported that a depressed battery of tests which included transferrin and albumin measurements, weight for height, and the midarm muscle circumference correlated with an increased incidence of infection and an increased mortality rate in a hospitalized population of veterans.[10] Similarly, Mullen et al. identified serum transferrin and albumin concentrations and anergy as prognostic indicators of postoperative morbidity and mortality in a surgical population.[11] Jensen et al. found low serum albumin and transferrin concentrations, a low total lymphocyte count, or anergy in response to a skin-test battery to predict subsequent infectious complications in orthopedic trauma patients.[12] The prognostic value of the serum transferrin concentration for predicting complications in a variety of clinical settings supports is routine inclusion in comprehensive nutritional evaluation.

METHOD

The serum transferrin concentration can be estimated directly by immunochemical methods or calculated indirectly from the total iron binding capacity. The technique of radial immunodiffusion (RID) has been developed for the precise quantitation of transferrin in plasma, utilizing antigen-antibody reactions in a gel matrix.[13] In the Mancini technique for RID, a protein antigen in solution is applied to a cylindrical well, and then diffuses radially into a thin gel matrix in which a monospecific antiserum is incorporated in uniform concentrations. The antigen applied to the RID plate is quantitated accurately by determining the diameter of the precipitin ring that forms when diffusion of the antigen has ceased, since the diameter of this ring is directly proportional to the amount of antigen applied.[14]

Because radial immunodiffusion is not routinely available for clinical use, serum transferrin is frequently calculated from measurements of the total iron binding capacity. Blackburn et al. have advanced a formula that has become commonly accepted for calculating the serum transferrin concentration[15,16]:

$$\text{Transferrin} = (\text{total iron binding capacity} \times 0.8) - 43.$$

This indirect calculation overestimates the transferrin concentration by

10 to 20 percent, since iron attaches to proteins other than transferrin when the latter is more than half saturated.[13] Several studies have cited discrepancies between transferrin concentrations as measured by RID and those derived from the TIBC.[17,18] Studies performed at the Miami Valley Hospital Burn Unit[18] found that although there is a mathematical relationship between the total iron binding capacity and serum transferrin levels, the conversion formula was different, as follows:

Serum transferrin = total iron binding capacity $\times$ 0.68 + 21.

Whether or not the burn injury was the independent variable is questionable. At any rate, modification of the formula institutionally may be necessary if clinically useful figures are to be obtained.

STANDARD/NORMAL RANGE

The average serum concentration of transferrin is about 295 mg/100 dl, and the normal adult range is 200 to 400 mg/dl. The normal adult range for TIBC is 250 to 350 mg/dl.[19]

DATA INTERPRETATION

Serum transferrin concentrations of less than 100 mg/dl are arbitrarily considered indicative of severe protein depletion, while concentrations between 100 and 200 mg/dl indicate marginal depletion and the need for further evaluation.[15]

Plasma concentrations of transferrin, like those of other serum proteins, are dependent not only on rates of synthesis but also on the utilization, intravascular transfer, catabolism, excretion and hydration.[19] Hypotransferrinemia of variable degree occurs in a variety of disorders, due either to impaired synthesis (e.g., cirrhosis, starvation, chronic infection) or increased excretion, as in the nephrotic syndrome.[19] Any acquired liver disease, particularly portal cirrhosis and hemochromatosis, may result in a diminished production of transferrin. Severe liver disease can result in marked depression of serum transferrin levels, with values as low as 60 mg/dl.[2] Similarly, serum transferrin levels are decreased with the anemia of chronic disease (hypochromic microcytic anemia).[1,20] Hypotransferrinemia is also encountered with chronic infection, neoplasia, iron overload, overhydration, renal disease, and other categories of chronic debilitating disease, as well as in excessive loss in nephrosis.[21] Protein-losing states, notably the nephrotic syndrome, can result in transferrin levels as low as 15 percent of normal.[2] Transferrin levels may be sharply depressed soon after thermal injury, and may remain low for up to 60 days.[22] In addition, serum transferrin concentration may be depressed by the administration of hormones or medications that inhibit protein synthesis, such as cortisone, L-asparginase, and testosterone.[23] Depressed serum transferrin levels have also been reported in zinc-deficient patients, which are corrected or improved with zinc supplementation.[24]

The value of serum transferrin determinations in detecting protein-calorie malnutrition is limited in the presence of iron deficiency anemia, which causes elevations in serum transferrin concentrations.

Increased levels of transferrin reflect the body's attempt to enhance its iron stores by issuing abundant amounts of iron-carrying protein, which serve to amplify iron absorption from the GI tract. Physiologic elevations of transferrin are seen with hypoxia and chronic blood loss, and during the second and third trimesters of pregnancy, and may be comparably induced by estrogen or oral contraceptive medications. Withdrawal of the medication or termination of pregnancy results in a return to normal concentrations.[23]

REFERENCES

1. Michiyasu, A. and Brown, E.B.: Studies of the metabolism of I-labeled human transferrin. J. Lab. Clin. Med. 61:363, 1963.
2. Ritchie, R.F.: Specific Proteins. In Clinical Diagnosis and Management by Laboratory Methods, 16th Ed. Henry, J.B. (ed.). W.B. Saunders Co., Philadelphia, 1979, pp. 242.
3. Ingelbleek, Y., Van Den Schrieck, H.G., DeNayer, P., et al.: Albumin, transferrin and the thyroxine-binding prealbumin/retinol binding protein (TBPA-RBP) complex in assessment of malnutrition. Clin. Chem. Acta 63:61, 1975.
4. Reeds, P.J. and Laditan, A.A.O.: Serum albumin and transferrin in protein-energy malnutrition: Their use in the assessment of marginal undernutrition and the prognosis of severe undernutrition. Br. J. Nutr. 36:255, 1976.
5. Young, G.A., Chem, C., and Hill, G.H.: Assessment of protein-calorie malnutrition in surgical patients from plasma proteins and anthropometric measurements. Am. J. Clin. Nutr. 31:429–435, 1978.
6. Shetty, P.S., Jung, R.T., Watraiewics, K.E., et al.: Rapid turnover transport proteins: An index of subclinical protein-energy malnutrition. Lancet: 230–232, 1979.
7. Kaminski, M.V., Fitzgerald, M.T., Murphy, R.J., et al.: Correlation of mortality with serum transferrin and anergy. JPEN 1:27, 1977.
8. Harvey, K.B., Ruggier, I.A., Regan, C.S., et al.: Hospital morbidity-mortality risk factors using nutritional assessment. Am. J. Clin. Nutr. 31:703, 1978.
9. Morath, M.A., Miller, S.F., and Finley, R.K.: Nutritional indicators of postburn bacteremic sepsis. JPEN 5:488, 1981.
10. Bienia, R., Ratcliff, S., Barbour, G.L., et al.: Malnutrition and hospital prognosis in the alcoholic patient. JPEN 6:301, 1982.
11. Mullen, J.L., Gertner, M.H., Buzby, G.P., et al.: Implications of malnutrition in the surgical patient. Arch. Surg. 114:121, 1979.
12. Jensen, J.E., Jensen, T.G., Smith, T., et al.: Nutrition and orthopaedics. J. Bone Joint Surg. 64A:1263, 1982.
13. Mardwitz, H. and Jiang, N.S.: Immunologic principles: The estimation and clinical significance of individual plasma proteins. In Fundamentals of Clinical Chemistry. Teiz, N. (ed.). W.B. Saunders Co., Philadelphia, 1976, Ch. 7.
14. M-Partigen Transferrin Kit Package Insert—Radial Immuno-diffusion Plates with Standard. Behring Diagnostics Division, American Hoechst Corporation, Somerville, N.J.
15. Blackburn, G.L., Bistrian, B.R., Maini, B.S., et al.: Nutritional and metabolic assessment of the hospitalized patient. JPEN 1:11, 1977.
16. Blackburn, G.L. and Thornton, P.A.: Nutritional assessment of the hospitalized patient. Med. Clin. North Am. 63:1103, 1979.
17. Rowlands, B.J., Jensen, T.G., and Dudrick, S.J.: Comparison of two methods of measurement of serum transferrin. JPEN 3:504, 1979.
18. Miller, S.F., Morath, M.A., and Finley, R.K.: Comparison of derived and

actual transferrin: A potential source of error in clinical nutritional assessment. J. Trauma 21:548, 1981.

19. Wallach, J.: Interpretation of diagnostic tests. In A Handbook Synopsis of Laboratory Medicine, 3rd Ed. Little Brown and Co., Boston, 1970.

20. Mancini, G., Carbonara, A.O., and Heremans, J.F.: Immunochemical quantitation of antigens by single radial immunodiffusion. Int. J. Immunochem. 2:235, 1965.

21. Jarnum, S. and Lassen, N.A.: Albumin and transferrin metabolism in infections and toxic diseases. Scand. J. Clin. Lab. Invest. 13:357, 1961.

22. Daniels, J.C., Cobb, E.K., Jones, J., et al.: Serum protein profiles in thermal burns. I. Serum electrophoretic patterns, immunoglobulins and transport proteins. J. Trauma 14:137, 1974.

23. Sher, P.P.: Drug interference with laboratory tests: Serum iron, iron binding capacity. Drug Therapy (Hosp): 30, July, 1977.

24. Bates, J. and McClain, C.J.: The effect of severe zinc deficiency on serum levels of albumin, transferrin and prealbumin in man. Am. J. Clin. Nutr. 34:1655, 1981.

F. Prealbumin and Retinol-Binding Protein _____

Prealbumin is known to transport about one-third of the active thyroid hormone, thyroxin, in the serum, and has accordingly been referred to as thyroxin-binding prealbumin (TBPA). In addition to this function in thyroxin transport, TBPA functions as a carrier protein for retinol-binding protein (RBP), the specific protein for vitamin A alcohol transport. Virtually all RBP is bound to prealbumin in a 1:1 ratio in the serum. It has been shown that the concentration of the TBPA-RBP complex decreases drastically in the acute stage of protein malnutrition and returns to normal during nutritional rehabilitation.[1-4]

Recently, investigators have evaluated prealbumin and retinol-binding protein as indicators of visceral protein status.[1-6] Because both of these proteins are very sensitive to short-term restrictions of protein and energy intake, and respond rapidly to refeeding, they are gaining increasing application as sensitive indicators of subclinical malnutrition and measures of the effectiveness of nutritional therapy. Both RBP and TBPA are much more responsive to dietary change than either transferrin or albumin. This sensitivity seems to be due to three factors: (1) biosynthesis of TBPA by the liver, which reacts promptly to protein deficiency; (2) the richness of TBPA in tryptophan and (3) the short half-lives of the two proteins.[2] In adult subjects the biological half-lives of TBPA and RBP are estimated at 2.5 to 3 days, and 12 hours, respectively.[3,7] Trypophan is known to exert a key role in the regulation of protein synthesis and is practically undetected in the blood of children with PCM.

The combination of their very rapid turnover rate and exceptionally high tryptophan content should explain why TBPA and RBP respond with marked sensitivity to protein depletion. However, because the two proteins strictly parallel one another in their behavior, determination of the prealbumin concentration has been recommended for routine clinical use, since this concentration is four to five times greater than that of RBP. Nevertheless, protein restriction does not have an immediate effect on the TBPA concentration if energy intake is maintained, since the synthesis of prealbumin is dependent upon both calorie and protein availability in the liver.[8] RBP is more sensitive, responding rapidly to protein and/or energy deprivation.[8] Therefore, both TBPA and RBP may prove helpful in the early diagnosis of subclinical malnutrition. These tests can also be used as indicators of protein synthesis during enteral or parenteral nutrition therapy, since the plasma levels of both respond within three days of treatment.[8] Additionally, the prealbumin level can be utilized as a test for visceral protein status in patients receiving exogenous albumin infusions.[9]

METHOD

Measurement of the plasma prealbumin and/or RBP concentration by radial immunodiffusion is simple, reproducible, accurate, and inexpensive. Radial immunodiffusion kits for the quantitation of RBP and prealbumin, based on the Mancini technique (see III D-Serum Transferrin), are available.[10]

STANDARDS/NORMAL RANGE

Quantitative analysis of the serum prealbumin concentration in normal adults yields values between 20 and 50 mg/100 ml, with a mean concentration of about 30 mg.[1,11] The normal adult human concentration of RBP is 3 to 6 μg/dl.[12]

DATA INTERPRETATION

Serum prealbumin and RBP concentrations of less than 10 mg/dl and 3 μg/dl respectively are indicative of visceral protein depletion. TBPA levels vary in various physiologic conditions (such as during pregnancy) and in various pathologic conditions, such as viral hepatitis and Laennec's cirrhosis.[1] Recent studies have indicated that prealbumin metabolism and clearance are independent of renal function.[13] Both concentrations are decreased in liver disease (cirrhosis, hepatitis), presumably due to interference with the normal liver functions of storage and synthesis. Levels are also decreased in hyperthyroidism and cystic fibrosis,[14,15] and low levels are common in stress, inflammation, and surgical trauma.[1] Metabolic studies with I-labeled TBPA indicate that a decreased synthesis is responsible for the depression of TBPA levels in acutely and chronically ill patients. Increased fractional TBPA degradation may also contribute to this depression.[1] The administration of corticoids results in an increase in serum prealbumin levels.[16]

All of these factors should be considered when interpreting transport protein values for nutritional assessment purposes.

REFERENCES

1. Ingenbleek, Y., DeVisser, M., and DeNayer, P.: Measurement of prealbumin as index of protein calorie malnutrition, Lancet 2:106, 1972.
2. Ingenbleek, Y., Van Den Schrieck, H.G., DeNayer, P., et al.: The role of retinol binding protein in protein-calorie malnutrition. Metabolism 24:633, 1975.

3. Ingenbleek, Y., Van Den Schrick, H.G., and DeNayer, P.: Albumin, transferrin and thyroxin-binding prealbumin/retinol-binding protein (TBPA-RBP) complex in assessment of malnutrition. Clin. Chim. ACTA 63:61, 1975.

4. Smith, F.R., Goodman, D.S., and Zaklama, M.S.: Serum vitamin A, retinol binding protein and prealbumin concentrations in protein calorie malnutrition: Functional defect in hepatic retinol release. Am. J. Clin. Nutr. 26:973, 1973.

5. Young, G.A. and Hill, G.L.: Evaluation of protein-energy malnutrition in surgical patients from plasma saline and other amino acids, proteins and anthropometric measurements. Am. J. Clin. Nutr. 34:166, 1981.

6. Smith, F.R., Suskind, R., Thanangkul, O. et al.: Plasma vitamin A, retinol-binding protein and prealbumin concentrations in protein-calorie malnutrition. III. Response to varying dietary treatments. Am. J. Clin. Nutr. 28:732, 1975.

7. Branch, W.T. Jr., Robbins, J., and Edelbach, H.: Thyroxine-binding prealbumin. J. Biol. Chem. 146:6011, 1971.

8. Shetty, P.S., Jung, R.T., Watraiewies, K.E., et al.: Rapid turnover transport proteins: An index of subclinical protein-energy malnutrition. Lancet 2:230, 1979.

9. Vanlandingham, S., Spiekerman, A.M., and Newmark, S.R.: Prealbumin: A parameter of visceral protein levels during albumin infusion. JPEN 6:230, 1982.

10. Mancini, G., Bargonna, A.O., and Heremans, J.F.: Immunological quantification of Antigens by Single Radial Immunodiffusion. Immunochemistry 2:235, 1965.

11. Kanda, Y., Goodman, D.S., Canfields, R.E., et al.: The amino acid sequence of human plasma prealbumin. J. Biol. Chem. 249:6796–605, 1974.

12. Haupt, H. and Heida, K.: Isoierung and Kristallisation des Retinol-Bindenden Proteins aus Human Serum. Blut 24:94–101, 1972.

13. Gofferje, H.: Prealbumin and retinol binding protein-highly sensitive parameters for the nutritional state in respect to protein. Medical Lab. 5:38–44, 1979.

14. Grant, A.: Laboratory assessment of nutrition states. In: Nutritional Assessment Guidelines. Cutter Medical 1979, pp. 36–39.

15. Smith, F.R., Underwood, B.A., Denning, C.R., et al: Depressed plasma retinol-binding protein levels in cystic fibrosis. J. Lab. Clin. Med. 80:423, 1972.

16. Ritchie, R.F.: Specific proteins. In Clinical Diagnosis and Management by Laboratory Methods, 16th Ed. Henry, J.B. (ed.). W.B. Saunders Co., Philadelphia, 1979, pp. 242.

G. Nitrogen Balance

CLINICAL SIGNIFICANCE

Because nitrogen is the primary component that differentiates protein from other basic nutrient modalities, the nitrogen balance is used as an index of protein nutritional status. The nitrogen balance may document the severity of catabolism in the unfed state or the degree of hypermetabolism, and provide data for serial monitoring of the adequacy of individualized nutritional support regimens.

The nitrogen balance represents the difference between nitrogen intake and output, this difference being positive during anabolism, negative during protein catabolism, and zero in nitrogen equilibrium. In normal healthy individuals, the rates of anabolism and catabolism are in equilibrium, thereby preserving the body protein mass and resulting in a nitrogen balance of zero. The nitrogen balance is negative when nitrogen excretion exceeds intake during accelerated protein catabolism (from major trauma or infection), or with the consumption of an inadequate diet. During pregnancy, growth, healing, or recovery from illness, when protein anabolism exceeds protein catabolism, the nitrogen balance is positive. The goal of supportive nutritional therapy is, of course, a positive nitrogen balance.[1,2]

METHOD

Ideally, determination of the nitrogen balance requires a meticulous evaluation of all routes of nitrogen intake (oral, enteral, parenteral) and of all routes of nitrogen excretion (urinary, fecal, dermal, and others). However, in the clinical setting these determinations are impractical if not impossible. Because urea accounts for 90 percent of the total urinary urea loss, and 90 to 95 percent of the daily nitrogen loss is excreted in the urine, the nitrogen balance can be computed[3-5] for clinical purposes as follows:

Nitrogen intake − (urine urea nitrogen + 4).

[Handwritten margin notes:]

$$\frac{Prot\ intake}{6.25} - $$

$$\left(\frac{N\ (g)}{urine\ (Ddl)} \cdot \frac{mg}{g} \times Total\ Urine\ (L) \cdot 24hr.\right)$$

$$+ 4g\ N$$

The latter factor accounts for stool and cutaneous loss as well as urinary nonurea nitrogen loss.[6] Urinary nonurea nitrogen losses are approximately 2 g/day, fecal losses are 1 g/day, and integumental losses (skin, hair, nails) are about 0.2 g/day in the average adult.[7] Thus, the factor of four is used to cover these losses.

To determine the nitrogen balance, the urinary urea nitrogen concentration is measured in milligrams per deciliter in an aliquot from a 24-hour urine specimen, is converted to grams per liter, and is multiplied by the total urine volume. The total number of grams of nitrogen excreted plus the factor of 4 grams is then subtracted from the total calculated nitrogen intake (protein intake ÷ 6.25) from all sources. When a 24-hour urine collection is not possible, a 12-hour urine collection can be used *if* the patient's nutrient intake is infused continuously over a 24-hour period. The amount of nitrogen excreted is then doubled. However, a 24-hour urine collection is mandatory for patients who have oral nutrient intake or who are receiving cyclic or intermittent infusions of enteral or parenteral solutions.[8]

DATA INTERPRETATION

The usual goal of nutritional therapy is to maintain the patient in a state of +4.0 to +6.0 g nitrogen balance. A negative nitrogen balance usually indicates accelerated protein catabolism, the consumption of an inadequate amount of protein, or insufficient calorie intake to provide energy requirements. Provision of adequate nitrogen and energy in a 1:150 grams of nitrogen to calorie ratio usually provides the basis for modification in nutritional therapy.

However, a nitrogen balance calculated by this method is invalid in patients with renal disease or urinary incontinence in whom urine excretion is impaired. In patients with renal disease, the urinary urea nitrogen excretion decreases and the blood urea nitrogen (BUN) concentration increases concurrently. Certain medications, such as methadone, may also interfere with urination. Additionally, because these calculations do not account for abnormal nitrogen losses, nitrogen excretion is underestimated in those patients with burns, diarrhea, vomiting, fistula drainage, or other abnormal nitrogen losses. The nitrogen-loss contribution from these sources is most difficult to estimate, since it is related to the size of injury and the amount of fluid drainage or loss. Therefore, in some clinical conditions, nitrogen losses are more difficult to quantify, and calculation of the nitrogen balance using a factor of 4 for nonurinary nitrogen losses will overestimate the balance.

REFERENCES

1. Munro, H.N. and Crim, M.C.: The proteins and amino acids. In Modern Nutrition in Health and Disease, 6th Ed. Goodhart, R.S. and Shils, M.S. (eds.). Philadelphia, Lea and Febiger, 1980.
2. Robinson, C.: Normal and Therapeutic Nutrition, 13th Ed. The Macmillan Co., New York, 1977.
3. Blackburn, G.L., Bistrian, B.R., Mani, B.S., et al.: Nutritional and metabolic assessment of the hospitalized patient. JPEN 1:11, 1979.

4. Harper, H., Rodwell, W., and Mayes, P.: Review of Physiological Chemistry. 16th Ed. Lange Medical Publications, Los Altos, CA, 1977.

5. Wilmore, D.: Metabolic Management of the Critically Ill. Plenum Medical Book Co., New York, 1977.

6. Mackenzie, T.A., Blackburn, G.L., and Flatt, J.P.: Clinical assessment of nutritional status using nitrogen balance. Fed. Proc. 33:63, 1974.

7. Sirba, E.: Effect of reduced protein intake on nitrogen loss from the human integumen. Am. J. Clin. Nutr. 20:1158, 1978.

8. Winborn, A.L., Banaszek, N.K., Freed, B.A., et al.: A protocol for nutritional assessment in a community hospital. J. Am. Diet. Assoc. 78:129, 1981.

H. Total Lymphocyte Count _____

Protein-calorie malnutrition is generally recognized as the most common cause of acquired immunodeficiency. Although numerous clinical observations and epidemiologic data document close association between protein-calorie malnutrition and increased susceptibility to infection, the exact relationship between nutrition and host defense mechanisms remains unclear. Host immunity is a complex interaction of three major systems: (1) cell-mediated immunity (the thymus dependent system often referred to as delayed hypersensitivity; (2) humoral antibody response (the apparent bone marrow dependent system); and (3) nonspecific immune responses which include phagocytosis and macrophage-mediated cytotoxicity.[1]

Cell-mediated immunity is an independent immune response mediated by a subset of lymphocytes commonly referred to as T cells. Before entering the lymphoid tissue or the blood, these cells undergo primary differentiation in the thymus, where their surfaces develop certain receptor sites that are specific for different antigens. Therefore, when foreign materials enter the body, lymphocytes bearing the appropriate receptor site will combine with them, initiating the delayed hypersensitivity response. Humoral immunity involves B lymphocytes which are characterized by membrane-bound immunoglobulins. When activated by an antigen, the B cells differentiate into immunoglobulin secreting cells. These antibodies comprise five immunoglobulin classifications: IgM, IgG, IgE, IgD, and IgA, each of which has a different function in the body. Included in the category of nonspecific immunity is phagocytosis, in which polymorphonuclears, leukocytes, and macrophages protect the host against invasion. Lysosomes discharged from granules within these cells and from complement are involved in destroying cellular bacteria. Although distinct, these three major systems are very interrelated and complex interactions between systems are additional determinants of host immunity.[1]

Although both antibody-producing capacity and cellular immunity are impaired by PCM, cellular immunity is affected earlier and more severely. With adult protein depletion, response to recall skin test antigens, total peripheral lymphocyte count, total thymus-derived cells, and in vitro response to antigens are reduced.[2,3] Adult marasmus has little effect on cellular immune function in terms of T lymphocytes, total lymphocytes or in vitro lymphocyte tests, although anergy to recall skin-test antigen is not unusual in patients who have experienced recent weight loss.[4]

The depressed total lymphocyte count has been correlated repeatedly with increased morbidity and mortality in hospitalized patients.[2,3,8-11] The preoperative TLC has been cited as a simple, reliable predictor of postoperative sepsis.[8] The TLC measured on the tenth postburn day has been identified as an index predictive of imminent septic episode in thermally injured patients.[10] Seltzer et al. reported that patients in an intensive care unit with depressed serum albumin levels and total lymphocyte counts had twice the complication rate and 4.5 times the mortality rate of those SICU patients with normal albumin levels and lymphocyte counts.[11] Because the TLC is closely associated with hypoalbuminemia, it is thought to be related to protein deficiency and amenable to correction with appropriate nutrition repletion.[2] Correlations between depressed total lymphocyte counts and impaired cell-mediated immunity have been established. Because the data for calculation of the total lymphocyte count are routinely obtained for most patients at admission, the total lymphocyte count has gained application as a screening indicator of immune and nutrition status.[12]

METHOD

The total lymphocyte count is calculated by multiplying the white blood cell count (WBC) by the differential for lymphocytes. The WBC is an absolute determination of total circulating leukocytes and expresses the number of WBCs in 1 microliter of blood as determined by automatic Coulter counting. This figure obtained must be multiplied by 1000 prior to calculation of total lymphocyte count. For example, a WBC count reported as 7.25 should be interpreted as 7250 WBCs per microliter of whole blood and this figure should be used in further calculations. The differential count is performed on a peripheral blood smear for identification of the different types of leukocytes and also identifies numbers of neutrophils, lymphocytes, monocytes, eosinophils, basophils and any abnormal cells as a percent of the total WBC count. Among the leukocytes, the neutrophils are usually the most abundant cells seen on a peripheral smear comprising 56 percent of the total white blood cell count. Normally 2.7 percent of cells will be eosinophils, 0.3 percent will be basophils, 7 percent will be monocytes, and 34 percent will be lymphocytes.[13]

STANDARDS/NORMAL RANGES

The normal WBC count is usually between 4500 and 11,000 cells/mm³ and may vary in a particular individual at different times during the day. The percent of lymphocytes in the differential usually varies between 20 percent and 35 percent. The normal range for the total lymphocyte count is generally accepted as between 2000 and 3500 cells per cubic millimeter.[14,15]

DATA INTERPRETATION

Significant lymphocytopenia has been defined as a total lymphocyte count of less than 1000 to 1200 cells/mm³, although a TLC of less than 1800 cells/mm³ indicates the need for further nutrition evaluation since some defect in immunocompetence may be present.

Factors other than malnutrition may cause or contribute to lymphocytopenia including injury, radiotherapy, and possibly surgery.[16-18] Additionally, the TLC is depressed by the administration of immunosuppressive medications such as steroids and chemotherapeutic agents.[16,19]

Similarly, the absolute value of the total lymphocyte count will be meaningless if the entire hematologic evaluation is not considered in data interpretation.[13] Specifically, the total lymphocyte count must be considered with the WBC since leukopenia or leukocytosis can cause errors in the interpretation of the TLC for purposes of evaluating nutrition status. Leukocytosis (elevated WBC) may be caused by a number of factors including tissue necrosis or infection. Usually leukocytosis increases with the severity of infection, and severe sepsis, tuberculosis, and nonmalignant infectious conditions may be associated with massive leukocytosis (termed the "Leukemoid Reaction"). The septic patient has a greatly increased number of neutrophils which may result in a very low percentage of lymphocytes. Chronic leukemia is also frequently characterized by a marked elevation in the leukocyte count. Relative lymphocytosis is a normal occurrence in infants and small children between four months and four years of age. In these situations, a normal or elevated TLC could be erroneously calculated in spite of malnutrition.[13]

Likewise, leukopenia (depressed WBC) can result in a low calculated total lymphocyte count in spite of normal nutrition status. Leukopenia may be caused by diminution of the WBC as a whole, decreases in neutrophils, or diminution of all blood elements. The following medications have been implicated in drug induced leukopenia: phenothiazides, antithyroid drugs, sulfonamides, phenylbutazone, chloramphenicol, phenindrone, corticosteroids, topical silver sulfadiazine, Temaril, Tagamet, Penicillin, Dalmane, and Lasix.[13,14,20] The presence of a large wound or burn may also result in a temporary depletion of peripheral lymphocytes in the serum due to tissue migration.[21] Leukopenia is also a frequent manifestation of viral infection.[13]

Therefore, the total lymphocyte count can be a sensitive indicator of immunocompetence and nutrition status only if prudently interpreted considering the other aspects of the hematological profile as well as the patient's status.

REFERENCES

1. Vitale, J.: Impact of nutrition on immune function. In: Nutrition and Disease, Ross Laboratories, Columbus, Ohio, 1979.
2. Bistrian, B.R., Blackburn, G.L., Scrimshaw, N.S., et al.: Cellular immu-

nity in semistarved states in hospitalized adults. Am. J. Clin. Nutr. 28:1148, 1975.

3. Law, D.K., Dudrick, S.J., and Abdou, N.I.: Immunocompetence in patients with protein-caloric malnutrition. Ann. Int. Med. 79:545, 1973.

4. Bistrian, B.R., Sherman, M., Blackburn, G.L., et al.: Cellular immunity in adult marasmus. Arch. Int. Med. 137:1408, 1977.

5. Guyton, A.: Basic Human Physiology: Normal Function and Mechanisms of Disease. Philadelphia: W.B. Saunders and Co., 1971.

6. Smythe, P.M., Schonland, M., and Brereton-Stiles, G.G., et al.: Thymolymphatic deficiency and depression of cell mediated immunity in protein caloric malnutrition, Lancet 2:939, 1971.

7. Dionigi, R., Zonta, A., Dominioni, L., et al.: The effects of total parenteral nutrition on immunodepression due to malnutrition. Ann. Surg. 185:467–474, 1977.

8. Lewis, R.T. and Klein, H.: Risk factors in postoperative sepsis: Significance of preoperative lymphocytopenia. J. Surg. Res. 26:365–371, 1975.

9. Harvey, K.B., Bothe, A., and Blackburn, G.L.: Nutritional assessment and outcome during oncologic therapy. Cancer 43:2065, 1975.

10. Morath, M.A., Miller, S.F., and Finley, R.K.: Nutritional indicators of postburn bacteremic sepsis. JPEN 5:488, 1981.

11. Seltzer, M.H., Fletcher, H.S., Seocum, B.A., et al.: Instant nutritional assessment in an intensive care unit. JPEN 5:70, 1981.

12. Seltzer, M.M., Bastidas, J.A., Cooper, D.M., et al.: Instant nutritional assessment. JPEN 3:157, 1979.

13. Tilkian, S.M., Conover, S.B., and Tilkian, A.G.: Routine hematology screening. In: Clinical Implications of Laboratory Tests. St. Louis, Missouri: C.V. Mosby Co., pp. 27–39, 1979.

14. Wallach, J.: Interpretation of Diagnostic Tests, 3rd Ed., Boston: Little Brown and Company, 1978.

15. Harrison's Principles of Internal Medicine, 6th Ed., New York: McGraw-Hill, 1970.

16. Copeland, E.M., MacFadyen, B.V., and Dudrick, S.J.: Effect of intravenous hyperalimentation on established delayed hypersensitivity in the cancer patient. Ann. Surg. 184:60–64, 1976.

17. Cosimi, A.B., Brunstetter, F.H., Kemmerer, W.T., et al.: Cellular immune competence of breast cancer patients receiving radiation therapy. Arch. Surg. 107:531, 1975.

18. Roth, J.A., Golub, S.H., Grimm, E.A., et al.: Effects of operation on immune response in cancer patients: Sequential evaluation of in vitro lymphocyte function. Surgery 79:46, 1976.

19. Hersh, E.M., Gutterman, J.U., Mavligit, G., et al.: Host defense, chemical immunosuppression and the transplant recipient: Relative effects of intermittent versus continuous immunosuppressive therapy with reference to objectives of treatment. Transplant Proc. 5:1191, 1973.

20. Physician's Desk Reference, 35th Ed., Oradell, NJ: Medical Economic Company, 1981.

21. Sakai, H., Daniels, J.C., Beathard, G.A., et al.: Mixed lymphocyte culture reactions in patients with acute thermal burns. J. Trauma 14:53, 1974.

I. Skin Antigen Testing

Failure of the immune system, particularly of cell-mediated immunity, has been documented in children and adults with moderate to severe malnutrition, both in developing countries and also in hospitalized patients in this country. Delayed cutaneous hypersensitivity (DCH) skin antigen testing is an inexpensive, convenient and widely available correlate of cell-mediated immunity which has been used extensively in hospitals to evaluate the cellular immune response of patients. A delayed reactive response at the antigen injection site indicates that the afferent, central, and efferent limbs of the immune response are intact and that the patient is capable of a nonspecific inflammatory response.[1]

Recent studies have documented failure of the delayed cutaneous response in malnourished hospitalized patients, with 5 to 50 percent of patients studied reported to be anergic to a battery of skin test antigens.[2-15] Repletion of body cell mass with intravenous hyperalimentation has been followed by restoration of skin reactivity[2,10] and the improvement of visceral protein status through nutritional repletion has been shown to reverse the effects of malnutrition on immune competence.[2-5,12]

Additionally, cutaneous anergy has been shown to be a significant risk factor for infection, sepsis and mortality in hospitalized patients with various clinical conditions,[14-21] mortality in the elderly[22] and a poor prognostic sign in a variety of malignant conditions.[23-26]

The anergic state has identified postoperative and posttrauma patients at increased risk for sepsis and mortality, and presaged these complications in patients studied preoperatively.[14-16] Serial testing of skin reactivity at weekly intervals has been reported as a sensitive guide to prognosis and adequacy of clinical management.[14] Anergy to a skin test battery has also been reported to predict imminent septic episodes in thermally injured patients when evaluated on the tenth postburn day.[17]

METHOD

Although the procedure for the application of skin test antigens (see Section II-O) is generally accepted and uniformly utilized, close scrutiny of methods for selecting antigen solutions and interpreting skin test responses is warranted and essential.

At this time, there is no uniform consensus of opinion regarding the selection of appropriate antigens for use in hospitalized patients. Several different protocols for skin antigen testing have been published to date. Blackburn, et al. uses streptokinase-streptodornase (SK-SD), mumps, and *Candida* antigens.[27] The standard battery of antigens applied by Winborn, et al. consists of SK-SD, mumps, *Candida*, and tuberculin purified protein derivative (PPD).[28] Dudrick, et al. apply this battery with the addition of trichophyton.[24] In order to select the minimum battery of appropriate antigens for skin testing, data are necessary on the response rates to each antigen and the minimum number and type of antigens required to determine anergy. Response rates to skin test antigens have been published for presumably normal populations, but few studies are available on hospitalized patients—a population of greater significance.[30,31] Palmer, et al. assessed delayed cutaneous hypersensitivity to 6 antigens in 752 predominantly male, general medical, surgical, neurological, and orthopedic inpatients at the Albuquerque Veterans Administration Hospital.[32] Reported response rates to the antigens were: mumps, 68 percent; *Candida*, 63 percent; trichophyton, 62 percent; tuberculin-PPD, 33 percent; histoplasmin, 26 percent; and coccidioidin, 13 percent. Half of the patients reacted concurrently to two of the first three antigens, and 92 percent reacted to at least one antigen. Since no single test was uniformly positive in the 92 percent of patients who responded to at least one antigen, it was concluded that a battery of tests was essential to determine anergy. This study did not include streptokinase-streptodornase, a commonly used antigen.[11]

In a review of 806 skin test applications at Hermann Hospital in Houston, Texas, 47 percent of readings were anergic while 53 percent of patients reacted to at least one antigen.[8] The number of reactive responses was greatest for streptokinase-streptodornase (30 percent) followed by mumps antigen (28 percent), trichophyton (20 percent), *Candida* (16 percent) and lastly PPD (9 percent). Streptokinase-streptodornase and mumps antigens together detected 82 percent of the reactive responders. The addition of trichophyton to this battery increased this figure to 94 percent, while the inclusion of *Candida* accounted for 97 percent of total reactive responders. The selection of antigens for routine use is further complicated by sporadic availability of certain antigens from manufacturers (e.g., streptokinase-streptodornase and mumps).

Considerable controversy also exists regarding the interpretation of a "positive" or reactive response to skin antigens. Although many investigators stipulate induration of at least 5 mm in diameter at 48 hours to any one antigen as sufficient evidence of intact immune responsiveness, the validity of this interpretation should be questioned. The package insert for mumps skin test antigen states that a positive reaction consists of 15 mm of erythema at 24 to 36 hours. Package inserts for tuberculin PPD, trichophyton, streptokinase-streptodornase, and *Candida* all stipulate induration of greater than 5 mm at 24 to 72 hours as a reactive response. Most subjects who are tested repeatedly exhibit accelerated reactions which start within several hours postinjection, peak within 24 hours and subside quite rapidly.[33] This phenomenon was described by Mantoux in 1912 and is particularly striking if the same site is used for serial testing.[34] Thus, 48 hour readings may often reflect substantially less than the peak response and occasionally give false-negative results because the reaction has already faded.

Results of the study in Houston indicate that skin test responses should be measured at both 24 and 48 hours postinjection and should be considered reactive or positive if induration $\geq$ 5 mm is noted at either time. Of these positive reactions, 19 percent of those for trichophyton occurred only at 24 hours postinjection and thus would have been read as negative if measured only at 48 hours postinjection. Similarly, 21 percent of the reactive responses to *Candida*, 16 percent to streptokinase-streptodornase, 28 percent to mumps, and 18 percent to PPD would have been recorded falsely negative if only 48 hour readings were considered. On the other hand, 22 percent of the reactive responses to trichophyton, 28 percent of those to *Candida*, 22 percent of those to streptokinase-streptodornase, 25 percent of those to mumps, and 30 percent of those to PPD would have been missed if reactions were measured only at 24 hours. Although the majority of reactions were positive at both 24 and 48 hours, a significant number of positive reactions to each antigen would be missed by measurement of either 24 or 48 hours exclusively.[8]

DATA INTERPRETATION

A positive or reactive reaction to a skin test antigen is interpreted as induration of 5 mm or greater at 24 to 72 hours postinjection. This cutaneous skin response is a cellular infiltration of mononuclear cells. The local vasodilation may also cause erythema or redness at this site but this response has no significance in the interpretation of delayed hypersensitivity reactions. The absence of any measurable area of induration is termed anergy. The term "relative anergy" has been applied to measurable induration of 1 to 4 mm during this time span to distinguish a suboptimal response from a nonresponse.

Patients who do not react to skin antigen testing may be malnourished since depressed visceral protein status as well as specific nutrient deficiencies have been associated with depression of the host's immune response and particularly cell-mediated immunity. However, many diseases, treatments, and other factors often present concurrently in malnourished populations may also suppress the cellular immune response and these effects must be noted in the interpretation of data.

A variety of infections including viral,[35-38] granulomatous,[39,40] and bacterial[35,36,39] have been shown to abrogate normal skin test responses. Other diseases associated with abnormal skin test responses include uremia,[41,42] cirrhosis,[43,44] hepatitis,[45,46] inflammatory bowel disease,[47,48] and sarcoid.[49,50] Anergy in cancer patients is also common, the frequency influenced by tumor histology, with squamous cancer and sarcoma patients experiencing depressed reactions more frequently than those with adenocarcinoma or melanoma.[51–53] Although most studies have found that an advancing stage of cancer is associated with worsening depression of DCH, abnormal skin test responsiveness is present even in early stages of many cancers.[54–56] The above mentioned disease states are also associated with a high incidence of protein-calorie malnutrition, and in clinical practice it is difficult to distinguish the effects of disease versus nutrition on cell-mediated immunity. However, the practitioner should be cognizant that anergy may be due to disease rather than malnutrition, particularly when other indicators of nutrition status improve consistently during nutrition therapy while anergy persists.

Disorders of the immune system will, of course, depress skin test reactivity; such disorders include congenital conditions such as Wiscott-Aldrich and DiGeorge's syndromes, and acquired conditions such as rheumatoid arthritis.[57,58] In addition, it appears that trauma and perhaps hemorrhage alone in the absence of malnutrition can temporarily produce anergy.[59,60] The early phase of thermal injury will also obliterate skin test reactivity independently of nutritional status.[61]

Many commonly used medications affect the skin test response including steroids,[62] immunosuppressants,[63] and chemotherapeutic agents.[64] Cimetidine,[65] coumadin,[66] and possibly aspirin[67] may also influence results. Therefore, concurrent medication therapy must also be taken into consideration when interpreting data on skin test reactions. Therapeutic doses of radiation therapy can also cause severe depression of cell-mediated immunity including anergy, although the duration of this effect is unknown.[68]

General anesthesia and/or operation has been found to alter skin test responses by most investigations.[69–71] In light of this data, skin test antigens should not be applied during the immediate postoperative period (48 hours) since the stress of surgery alone will complicate the valid interpretation of results.

Additionally, the inflammatory response when assessed by skin reactivity is diminished in iron and zinc deficiency states. Although the mechanism is unclear, restoration of reactive responses is followed by iron or zinc repletion.[72]

REFERENCES

1. Edelman, R.: Cell-mediated immune response in protein-caloric malnutrition—a review. In Malnutrition and the Immune Response, Suskind, RM (ed), New York: Raven Press, 1977.
2. Law, D.K., Dudrick, S.J., and Abdou, N.I.: Immunocompetence of patients with protein-caloric malnutrition. The effects of nutritional repletion. Ann. Intern. Med. 79:545, 1973.
3. Bistrian, B.R., Blackburn, G.L., Scrimshaw, N.S., et al.: Cellular immunity in semistarved states in hospitalized adults. Am. J. Clin. Nutr. 28: 1148, 1975.

4. Bistrian, B.R., Sherman, M., Blackburn, G.L., et al.: Cellular immunity in adult marasmus. Arch. Intern. Med. 137:1408, 1977.
5. Blackburn, G.L., Gibbons, G.W., Bothe, A., et al.: Nutritional support in cardiac cachexia. J. Thorac. Cardiovasc. Surg. 73:489, 1977.
6. Jensen, J.E., Smith, T.K., Jensen, T.G., et al.: Nutritional assessment of orthopaedic patients undergoing total hip replacement surgery—the Frank Stinchfield Award paper. In The Hip, St. Louis, Missouri: C.V. Mosby, 1981.
7. Jensen, J.E., Jensen, T.G., Smith, T.K., et al.: Nutrition in orthopedic surgery. Orthopaedic Transactions 5:447, 1981.
8. Jensen, T.G., Englert, D.M., Dudrick, S.J., et al.: Delayed hypersensitivity in skin testing: Response rates in a surgical population. J. Am. Dietet. A. (in press).
9. Jensen, J.E., Smith, T.K., Jensen, T.G., et al.: Nutrition in orthopedic surgery. J. Bone. and Joint Surg., (in press).
10. Copeland, E.M., MacFadyen, B.V., and Dudrick, S.J.: Effect of intravenous hyperalimentation on established delayed hypersensitivity in the cancer patient. Ann. Surg. 184:60, 1976.
11. Daly, J.M., Dudrick, S.J., and Copeland, E.M.: Evaluation of nutritional indices as prognostic indicators in the cancer patient. Cancer 43:925, 1979.
12. Spanier, A.H., Meakins, J.L., MacLean, L.D., et al.: The relationship between immune competence and nutrition. Surg. Forum 27:332, 1976.
13. Meakins, J.L., Christou, N.V., Halle, C.C., et al.: Influence of cancer on host resistance and susceptibility to infection. Surg. Forum 30:115, 1979.
14. Willcutts, H.D., Linderme, D., Chlastawa, D., et al.: Anergy: Is nutritional reveral possible/outcome significant? JPEN 3:292, 1979.
15. Meakins, J.L., Pietsch, J.B., Bubenick, O., et al.: Delayed hypersensitivity: Indicator of acquired failure of host defenses in sepsis and trauma. Ann. Surg. 186:241, 1977.
16. MacLean, L.D., Meakins, J.L., Taguchi, K., et al.: Host resistance in sepsis and trauma. Ann. Surg. 182:207, 1975.
17. Morath, M.A., Miller, S.F., Finley, R.K.: Nutritional indicators of postburn bacteremic sepsis. JPEN 5:488, 1981.
18. Dionigi, P., Nazari, S., Bonoldi, A.P., et al.: Nutritional assessment and surgical infections in patients with gastric cancer or peptic ulcer. JPEN 6:128, 1982.
19. Biena, R., Ratcliff, S., Barbour, G.L., et al.: Malnutrition and hospital prognosis in the alcoholic patient. JPEN 6:301, 1982.
20. Kaminski, M.V., Fitzgerald, M.T., Murphy, R.J., et al.: Correlation of mortality with serum transferrin and anergy. JPEN 1:27, 1979.
21. Buzby, G.P., Muller, J.L., Mathews, D.C., et al.: Prognostic nutritional index in gastrointestinal surgery. Am. J. Surg. 139:160, 1980.
22. Roberts, Thompson, I.C., Whittingham, S., and Youngchaiyud, U.: Aging, immune response and mortality. Lancet 2:368, 1970.
23. Hersh, E.M., Gutterman, J.V., Mavligit, G.M., et al.: Serial studies of immunocompetence of patients undergoing chemotherapy for acute leukemia. J. Clin. Invest. 54:401, 1974.
24. Israel, L., Mugica, J., Chahinian, P.: Prognosis of early bronchogenic carcinoma. Survival curves of 451 patients after rejection of lung cancer in relation to results of preoperative tuberculin skin test. Biomed. 19:68, 1973.
25. Eilber, E.R. and Morton, D.L.: Impaired immunologic reactivity and recurrence following cancer surgery. Cancer 25:363, 1970.
26. Sokol, J.E. and Aungst, C.W.: Response to BCG vaccination and survival in advanced Hodgkin's disease. Cancer 24:128, 1969.
27. Blackburn, G.L., Bistrian, B.R., Mani, B.S., et al.: Nutritional and metabolic assessment of the hospitalized patient. J. Parent. Ent. Nutr. 1:11, 1979.

28. Winborn, A.L., Banazek, N.K., and Freed, B.A.: A protocol for nutritional assessment in a community hospital. J. Am. Dietet. Assoc. 78:129, 1981.

29. Dudrick, S.J., Jensen, T.G., and Rowlands, B.J.: Nutritional support: Assessment and indications. In Nutrition in Clinical Surgery, Deitel, M. (ed): 1979.

30. Angle, R.M.: The use of mumps skin test in adults. JAMA 177:650, 1961.

31. Shannon, D.C., Johnson, G., Rosen, F.S., et al.: Cellular reactivity to *Candida albicans* antigen. N. Engl. J. Med. 275:690, 1966.

32. Palmer, D.L. and Reed, W.P.: Delayed hypersensitivity skin testing. Response rates in a hospital population. J. Inf. D. 130:132, 1974.

33. Sokal, J.E.: Measurement of delayed skin test responses. N. Engl. J. Med., 293:501, 1975.

34. Mantoux, Ch.: La boie intradermique en tuberculine-therapie. Presse Med., 20:146, 1912.

35. Mitchell, A.G., Nelson, W.E., and LeBlanc, T.J.: Studies in immunity V. effect of acute diseases on the reaction of the skin to tuberculin. Am. J. Dis. Child 49:695, 1935.

36. Westwater, J.S.: Tuberculin allergy in acute infectious diseases. Quart. J. Med. 4:203, 1935.

37. Reed, W.P., Olds, J.W., and Kisch, A.L.: Decreased skin test reactivity associated with influenza. J. Infect. Dis. 125:398, 1972.

38. Mangi, R.J., Niederman, J.C., Kelleher, J.E., et al.: Depression of cell-mediated immunity during acute infectious mononucleosis. N. Engl. J. Med. 291:1149, 1974.

39. Turk, J.L. and Walters, M.F.R.: Cell-mediated immunity in patients with leprosy. Lancet 2:243, 1969.

40. Bullock, W.E.: Studies on immune mechanisms in leprosy. N. Engl. J. Med. 278:298, 1974.

41. Wilson, W.E.C., Kirkpatric, C.H., and Talmage, D.W.: Suppression of immunologic responsiveness in uremia. Ann. Int. Med. 62:1–14, 1965.

42. Bansal, V.K., Popli, S., Pickering, J., et al.: Protein-caloric malnutrition and cutaneous anergy in hemodialysis maintained patients. Am. J. Clin. Nutr. 33:1608, 1980.

43. Straus, B., Berenyi, M., Ming-Huang, J., et al.: Delayed hypersensitivity in alcoholic cirrhosis. Dig. Dis. 16:509, 1971.

44. Fox, R.A., Scheuer, P.J., Sherloch, S., et al.: Impaired delayed hypersensitivity in primary biliary cirrhosis. Gut 9:729, 1968.

45. Snyder, N., Bessoff, J., Dwyer, J.M., et al.: Depressed delayed cutaneous hypersensitivity in alcoholic hepatitis. Dig. Dis. 23:353, 1978.

46. Toh, B.H., Roberts-Thomson, I.C., Mathew, J.D., et al.: Depression of cell mediated immunity in old age and the immunopathic diseases, lupus erythematosis, chronic hepatitis and rheumatoid arthritis. Clin. Exp. Immunol. 14:193, 1973.

47. Thayer, W.R., Fixa, B., Komarkova, O., et al.: Skin test reactivity in inflammatory bowel disease in the United States and Czechoslovakia, Dig. Dis. 23:337, 1978.

48. Sashar, D.B., Taub, R.N., Ramachandar, K., et al.: T and B lymphocytes and cutaneous anergy in inflammatory bowel disease. Ann. N.Y. Acad. Sci. 278:565, 1976.

49. Goldstein, R.A., Janicki, B.W., Mirro, J., et al.: Cell-mediated immune responses in sarcoidosis. Am. Rev. Resp. Dis. 117:55, 1978.

50. Chusid, E.L., Shah, R., and Siltzback, L.E.: Tuberculin tests during the course of sarcoidosis in 350 patients. Am. Rev. Resp. Dis. 104:13, 1971.

51. Bolton, P.M., Mander, A.M., Davidson, J.M., et al.: Cellular immunity in cancer: Comparison of delayed hypersensitivity skin tests in three common cancers. Br. Med. J. 3:18–20, 1975.

52. Chretien, P.B., Catalona, W.J., Twomey, P.L., et al.: Correlation of

immune reactivity and clinical status in cancer. Ann. Clin. Lab. Sci. 4:331, 1974.

53. Pinsky, C.M., Oettgen, H.F., El Domeiri, A., et al.: Delayed hypersensitivity reactions in patients with cancer. Proc. Am. Assoc. Cancer Res. 12:100, 1971.

54. Turnbull, A.R., Turner, D.T.L., and Fraser, J.B.: Anergy—a prognostic indicator in early breast cancer. Br. Med. J. 2:932, 1978.

55. Solowey, A.C. and Rapaport, F.T.: Immunologic responses in cancer patients. Surg. Gynecol. Obstet. 121:756, 1965.

56. Eilber, F.R., Nizze, J.A., and Morton, D.L.: Sequential evaluation of general immune competence in cancer patients: correlation of clinical course. Cancer 35:660, 1975.

57. Spitler, L.E.: Delayed hypersensitivity skin testing. In Manual of Clinical Immunology, Rose, N.R. and Friedman, H. (eds): Washington, D.C.: American Society for Microbiology, 1976, pp. 53-63.

58. Andrianakos, A.A., Sharp, J.T., Person, D.A., et al.: Cell-mediated immunity in rheumatoid arthritis. Ann. Rheum. Dis. 36:13–20, 1977.

59. Meakins, J.L., MacLean, A.P., Kelly, R., et al.: Delayed hypersensitivity and neutrophil chemotaxis: Effect of trauma. J. Trauma 18:240, 1978.

60. Pietsch, J.B., Meakins, J.L., and MacLean, L.D.: The delayed hypersensitivity response: Application in clinical surgery. Surgery 82:349, 1977.

61. Aiebert, J.M., McGough, M., Rodehearer, G., et al.: The influence of catabolism on immunocompetence in burned patients. Surgery 86:242, 1979.

62. Bovornkitti, S., Knsadal, P., Sathirapat, P., et al.: Reversion and reconversion rate of tuberculin skin reactions in correlation with the use of prednisone. Dis. Chest 38:51, 1960.

63. Maibach, H. and Epstein, L.: Immunologic responses in healthy volunteers receiving azathioprine (Imuran). Int. Arch. Allergy 27:102, 1965.

64. Boeva, M., Donchev, T., Markova, R., et al.: Delayed hypersensitivity reactions in patients with breast cancer. Neoplasm 25:733, 1978.

65. Goodwin, J.S.: Cimetidine and delayed hypersensitivity (letter). Lancet 1:934, 1978.

66. Edwards, R.L. and Rickles, F.R.: Delayed hypersensitivity in man: Effects of systematic anticoagulation. Science 200:541, 1978.

67. Yazici, H., Saville, P.D., and Chaperon, E.D.: Aspirin suppression of delayed hypersensitivity. Clin. Res. 22:645, 1974.

68. Wara, W.M., Phillips, T.L., Wara, D.W., et al.: Immunosuppression following radiation therapy for carcinoma of the nasopharynx. Am. J. Roentgenol. 123:482, 1975.

69. Bruce, D.L. and Wingard, D.W.: Anesthesia and the immune response. Anesthesiology 34:271, 1971.

70. Tarpley, J.L., Twomey, P.L., Catalona, W.J., et al.: Suppression of cellular immunity by anesthesia and operation. J. Surg. Res. 22:195, 1977.

71. Park, S.K., Brody, J.I., Wallace, A.A., et al.: Immunosuppressive effect of surgery. Lancet 1:53, 1971.

72. Strauss, R.G.: Iron deficiency, infections and immune function: A reassessment. A. J. Clin. Nutr. 31:660, 1978.

J. Nutritional Diagnosis _____

Nutrition diagnoses are classified as marasmus, kwashiorkor, and marasmus/kwashiorkor or severe protein-calorie malnutrition, in accordance with criteria cited in the International Classification of Diseases. Although kwashiorkor and marasmus represent the two major classifications of malnutrition, combinations and degrees of both exist. Depression of any index or measurement may indicate or substantiate the need for aggressive nutritional intervention when the patient's clinical condition, nutrient requirements and clinical treatment are carefully considered.

Adult marasmus or chronic inanition is characterized by depressed anthropometric measurements in the presence of normal serum protein concentrations, and is usually manifested by prolonged, gradual wasting of subcutaneous fat and skeletal muscle mass secondary to inadequate nutrient intake or malabsorption. Marasmic individuals may often be identified by visual inspection and this condition is common in those patients with cancer and other chronic illnesses.

Adult kwashiorkor or protein depletion is common in the patient with a combination of severe catabolic stress and low nutrient intake. Trauma patients and those with major burns frequently exhibit this syndrome. Due to the rapidity of onset, these patients often maintain normal anthropometric measurements despite severe depression of serum protein concentrations and impaired immunocompetence. Edema is also a common feature due to hypoalbuminemia and altered electrolyte metabolism.

Marasmic/kwashiorkor like malnutrition is regarded as the advanced stage of protein-calorie malnutrition. This is a life-threatening situation characterized by a high incidence of nutritionally related complications. It occurs most commonly in patients who have mobilized fat and lean body mass for prolonged periods in an unsuccessful

TABLE 12. BASAL ENERGY EXPENDITURE (BEE)

HARRIS-BENEDICT EQUATION

Men

$$BEE = 66 + (13.7 \times W) + (5 \times H) - (6.8 \times A)$$

Women

$$BEE = 655 + (9.6 \times W) + (1.7 \times H) - (4.7 \times A)$$

W = actual weight in kg; H = height in cm; A = age in yr.

effort to recover from chronic disease or severe injury. Ultimately these reserves are depleted and rapid depression of visceral protein synthesis supervenes. Clinically the appearance of hypoalbuminemic edema, decline in immunocompetence and evidence of deterioration in the function of multiple organ systems signal its occurrence. Vigorous nutritional therapy is obviously essential.

ASSESSMENT OF INDIVIDUAL ENERGY/NUTRIENT REQUIREMENTS

In addition to initial determination of the presence and degree of nutritional depletion, an estimation of individual energy and protein requirements is essential for planning nutritional management. Energy needs of normal individuals are ordinarily considered to be the sum of basal energy expenditure, the calories expended for physical activity and a small increment for the specific dynamic action of food. Basal energy expenditure can be reasonably calculated from the Harris-Benedict Equation for men and women (Table 12). Based on age, sex, height and weight, this equation more accurately reflects caloric requirements than methods using weight alone.

Long, et al. compared predicted BMR values calculated from the Harris-Benedict equation to measured values by gas analyzer and found only a 2.9 percent difference in the two values.[2] The standards of Boothby, et al.[3] or Fleish[4] may also be used to calculate BMR. Wilmore[5] has stated that those of Fleish represent the best standards. However, the high correlation between BMR calculated by the Harris-Benedict equation and measured values obtained by gas analyzer[2] indicate that this calculation represents an accurate evaluation of BMR.

In the hospitalized patients estimates of total caloric need must also include additional energy expenditure for physical activity, the specific dynamic action of food and stress (surgery, fever, sepsis, trauma). The patient who sits beside the bed may increase daily energy expenditure 5 to 10 percent above basal rates and the majority of ambulatory patients expend no more than 20 percent above basal rates for physical activity.[6] Long, et al. converted activity figures to calories expended for a group of patients while sitting, standing and walking.[7] During a 24-hour period, when a patient was supine 50 to 80 percent of the time and spent less than 10 percent of the day walking, preoperative caloric activity requirements were approximately 20 percent greater than resting values. The first postoperative period (4 days) was increased by only 5 percent, the second 4 days by 10 percent, and the third 15 percent. The specific dynamic action of ingested food is calculated at approximately 10 percent of consumed calories but failure to account for this effect is a small error in hypermetabolic or critically ill patients, since a smaller quantity of energy production following food ingestion is observed.[6]

Extensive studies on critically ill surgical patients utilizing a continuous gas analyzer for expired air analysis and nitrogen excretion measurements have established ranges for estimating the increase in basal energy expenditure above normal levels during injury or stress. General increases above basal metabolic expenditure have been reported for patients with multiple fractures, sepsis, burns and also following elective surgical operation.[7-10] This increase in metabolic requirements may range from 10 percent in the patient undergoing surgery without complication to 125 percent above predicted normal values following major thermal burn. Energy requirements can be estimated with increases for these conditions using a nomogram published by Wilmore[5] (Figure 1). Total daily caloric requirements can also be calculated using the Harris-Benedict equation and adjusting this value upward using activity and injury factors reported by Long to estimate total energy requirements[2] (Figure 2). A simple method for estimating caloric requirements is to supply calories at 35 cal/kg/day for maintenance and 45 kcal/kg/day for anabolism.[11] Rutten, et al. suggested caloric intakes may be calculated by multiplying basal energy expenditure by 1.76 to 2.0 for mild to moderate catabolic states.[12] Since caloric requirements following thermal injury are directly proportional to the extent of burn injury, several investigators have reported formulas for calculating energy requirements for these patients which are based on burn size. Curreri[13] suggests 25 kcal × kg body weight + 40 kcal × % burn, while Sutherland[14] recommends 20 kcal body weight + 70 kcal × % burn. The calculations mentioned above will only provide estimates of energy requirements for individual patients, and careful monitoring of actual energy intake and weight change is warranted during nutritional intervention to provide guidelines for further modification of therapy.

The normal man engaging in an average amount of exercise requires 0.5 to 1.0 g protein/kg each day. In the moderately stressed individual (i.e., with infection, fracture, major surgery), protein requirements increase to 1.5 to 2.0 g/kg, and the severely stressed individual (with burns, major trauma) may require 2.0 to 4.0 mg/kg each day to establish positive nitrogen balance. A gram of nitrogen to a caloric ratio of 1:150 is adequate for most catabolic patients, although lower ratios may be desirable in renal disease and higher ratios during severe stress. Protein requirements per day can be calculated as follows:[10,15]

$$\text{Protein (g)} = \frac{6.25 \times \text{calorie requirements}}{150}$$

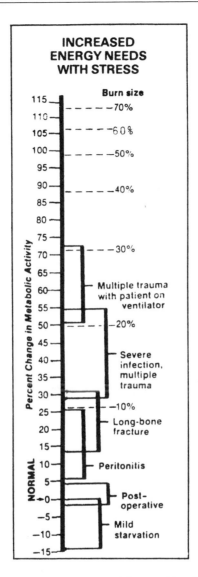

Figure 1. Increased Energy Needs with Stress nomogram. (Adapted from Wilmore, D.: The Metabolic Management of the Critically Ill. New York, Plenum, 1977.)

However, a more realistic evaluation of protein requirements might be ascertained by measuring urea nitrogen in a 24-hour urine specimen. In most instances this will represent over 85 percent of the N loss in a 24-hour urine sample and may be adjusted to total N by dividing by 0.85.[2]

Most calculated increases above resting requirements are estimates based upon maximum mean values measured in various groups of patients. Therefore, it is necessary to make adjustments in intakes of calories and N during the period of convalescence, since requirements

Figure 2. Estimating Caloric Requirements.

Male:

$[66 + 13.7 \,(W) + 5 \,(H) - 6.8 \,(A)] \times AF \times IF$

Female:

$[665 + 9.6 \,(W) + 1.85 \,(H) - 4.7 \,(A)] \times AF \times IF$

AF = Activity Factor		*IF = Injury Factor*	
Confined to bed	1.2	Minor operations	1.20
Ambulatory	1.3	Skeletal trauma	1.35
		Major sepsis	1.60
		Severe thermal burn	2.10

Sample Calculations:

Female: *Caloric Requirements*

$[665 + 9.6 \,(W) + 1.85 \,(H) - 4.7 \,(A)] \times AF \times IF$
$[665 + 9.6 \,(55 \text{ kg}) + 1.85 \,(163 \text{ cm}) - 4.7 \,(26 \text{ yr})] \times 1.2 \times 1.35$
$[665 + 528 + 302 - 122] \times 1.2 \times 1.35 = 2224 \text{ calories}$

Female: *Protein Requirements*

$2224 \div 150$ (n:Kcal ratio) $= 14.8$ g nitrogen
14.8×6.25 (conversion factor) $= 93$ g protein

Male: *Caloric Requirements*

$[66 + 13.7 \,(W) + 5 \,(H) - 6.8 \,(A)] \times AF \times IF$
$[66 + 13.7 \,(70 \text{ kg}) + 5 \,(180 \text{ cm}) - 6.8 \,(32)] \times 1.2 \times 1.35$
$[66 + 959 + 1925 - 352.5] \times 1.2 \times 1.35 = 2765 \text{ calories}$

Male: *Protein Requirements*

$2765 \div 150$ (n:Kcal ratio) $= 18.4$ g nitrogen
18.4×6.25 (conversion factor) $= 115$ g protein

W = actual weight in kg, H = height in cm, A = age in yr. (From Long, et al.: Metabolic response to injury and illness. Estimation of energy and protein needs from indirect calorimetry and nitrogen balance. JPEN 3:452–456, 1979, with permission.)

for injury subside with time and healing. The adjustment in protein requirements can be easily ascertained by measuring urea nitrogen in a 24-hour urine sample on a serial basis. Caloric adjustments can then be made to maintain a calorie:N ratio of 150:1. Additionally, weight and caloric intake should be monitored daily to indicate caloric requirements.

REFERENCES

1. Harris, J.A. and Benedict, F.G.: Biometric studies of basal metabolism in man. Carnegie Institute of Washington, Publication #279, 1919.
2. Long, C.L., Schaffel, N., Geiger, J.W., et al.: Metabolic response to injury and illness: Estimation of energy and protein needs from indirect calorimetry and nitrogen balance. JPEN 3:452, 1979.
3. Boothby, W.M., Berkson, J., and Dunn, H.L.: Studies of the energy metabolism of normal individuals. Standard for basal metabolism with nomogram for clinical application. Am. J. Physiol. 116:468, 1936.
4. Fleisch, A.: Le métabolisme basal standard et sa détermination au moyen du "Metabocalculator". Helvet. Med. Acta 18:23, 1951.
5. Wilmore, D.W.: The metabolic management of the critically ill. King, T., Reemtsma, K. (eds), New York: Plenum Medical Book Co., 1977, p. 818.
6. Kinney, J.M.: Energy requirements of the surgical patient. In Ballinger, W.F., Collins, J.A., Ducker, W.R., Dudrick, S.J., and Zeppa, R. (eds), Manual of Surgical Nutrition, Philadelphia: W.B. Saunders Co., pp. 223–235, 1973.
7. Kinney, J.M., Duke, J.H., Long, C.L., et al.: Tissue fuel and weight loss after injury. J. Clin. Path. 23 (Suppl 4):65, 1970.
8. Kinney, J.M.: Energy deficits in acute illness and injury. In Proceedings of the Conference on Energy: Metabolism and Body Fuel Utilization. Morgon, A.P. (ed), Cambridge, Massachusetts: Harvard University Printing Office, p. 173, 1966.
9. Long, C.L.: Energy balance and carbohydrate metabolism in infection and sepsis. Am. J. Clin. Nutr. 30:1301, 1977.
10. Kinney, J.M., Long, C.L., Gump, F.E., et al.: Tissue composition of weight loss in surgical patients in elective operation. Ann. Surg. 168:459, 1968.
11. Copeland, E.M., Daly, J.M., and Dudrick, S.J.: Nutritional concepts in the treatment of head and neck malignancies. Head and Neck Surg., 350–363, 1969.
12. Rutten, P., Blackburn, G.L., Flatt, J.P., et al.: Determination of optimal hyperalimentation rate. J. Surg. Res. 18:477, 1975.
13. Curreri, P.W., Richmond, D., Marvin, J., et al.: Dietary requirements of patients with major burns. J. Am. Dietet. Assoc. 65:415, 1974.
14. Sutherland, A.B.: Nitrogen balance and nutritional requirements in the burn patient: A reappraisal. Burns 2:238, 1976.
15. Long, C.L., Crosby, F., Geiger, J.W., et al.: Parenteral nutrition in the septic patient: Nitrogen balance, limiting plasma, amino acids and calorie to nitrogen ratio. Am. J. Clin. Nutr. 29:380, 1976.

K. Modalities of Nutritional Support _____

Individual nutrient requirements are considered with initial metabolic and biochemical data to formulate the most appropriate nutritional therapy for each patient. When enteral alimentation is indicated, the most appropriate feeding method is selected by first determining the maximum number of calories and the amount of protein voluntarily ingested via the oral route over a 24-hour period. A nutritional supplement may be ordered to augment intake when conventional foods and beverages do not provide nutrient requirements. These requirements may be normal (as in patients with mastication or deglutition problems) or increased (as in sepsis, burns, or multiple trauma). A supplement is usually a commercially formulated liquid or powder containing one or more nutrients in a concentrated form. Some supplements may be ingested as between-meal foods or beverages to increase nutrient density. Modular supplements provide a source of a single nutrient (carbohydrate, protein, and/or fat) and may be mixed with food, beverages or other liquid formulas to increase intake of that nutrient.

Meal replacements are commercial formulas designed to provide adequate maintenance nutrition in a form compatible with tube administration. However, many formulas are flavored for oral consumption. Meal replacements usually provide approximately 35 percent of calories from fat sources and 12 to 16 percent from protein sources. Products vary considerably in osmolality, lactose, vitamin and mineral content, but in calorically adequate volumes, these formulas meet or exceed the Recommended Dietary Allowances for all nutrients. These products require intact digestive and absorptive processes and are indicated for those patients with adequate gastrointestinal function who cannot or will not consume foods and/or supplements in necessary quantities to meet nutrient requirements. Possible indications for meal replacements include: chewing or swallowing difficulties (i.e., cancer in throat or oral cavity, surgery or trauma to mouth and/or throat, mandibular fractures, stroke or paralysis), elevated nutrient requirements, or feeding by gastrostomy or jejunostomy to bypass upper gastrointestinal lesions, fistulas, or obstructions. Adherence to defined protocols and procedures is essential to administer tube feeding without complications.

Defined formula diets is a term used to designate nutritionally complete, chemically formulated powders that provide an easily digested liquid diet when mixed with water. Most defined formula diets are clear liquid, minimal in residue, and lactose-free. Ingredients may include amino acids, hydrolyzed protein, polysaccharides, oligosaccharides, essential fatty acids, vitamins and minerals. These nutrients require minimal digestion and are readily absorbed. However, comparative studies assessing the effectiveness of various preparations available remain to be done.

Defined formula diets may be indicated for nutritionally depleted patients who require preoperative bowel preparation, patients with gastrointestinal tract exfoliation associated with chemotherapy, and patients undergoing abdominal irradiation. Defined formula diets may also be indicated for patients who are unable to tolerate intact nutrients due to partial obstruction, short bowel syndrome, and chronic pancreatitis.

Clinical indications for intravenous hyperalimentation can be defined when adequate enteral intake is impossible, improbable, inadvisable or hazardous, and where specific metabolic requirements might be better met by intravenous rather than oral or enteral techniques. Examples of the latter include bowel obstruction, prolonged ileus, acute inflammatory bowel disease, hemorrhagic pancreatitis, short-gut syndrome, congenital anomalies, burns or other disorders resulting in massive catabolism.

However, selection of the most appropriate nutrition therapy for each patient must be based on consideration of individual metabolic and biochemical data, nutrient requirements, and capabilities. The willing and knowledgeable clinical dietitian can make a significant contribution to patient care by providing professional expertise in this decision-making process.

Index _____

207